Breast Cancer

and

Prostate Cancer

Avoidance &

Survival Guide

Simple, natural, money-saving, and drug-free ways to avoid and even reverse two of the most dreaded cancers

by
Robert Bernardini, M.S.

This publication is designed to provide accurate and authoritative information in regard to the subject matter covered. It is sold with the understanding that the publisher is not engaged in rendering medical, legal, or other professional services. If such advice or other expert assistance is required, the services of a competent professional person should be sought.

The ideas and suggestions contained in this book are not intended as a substitute for the appropriate care of a licensed health care practitioner. Qualified medical assistance should always be sought before beginning any treatments. The following is intended for educational purposes only and has not been evaluated by the FDA. Suggestions are not made to treat a specific condition.

Bernardini, Robert.
   Breast cancer and prostate cancer avoidance & survival guide/ by
   Robert Bernardini.
p.cm.
Includes bibliographical references
LCCN: 2010940661
ISBN: 97809703269-8-0

1. Health –Popular works. 2. Medicine, Preventive—
Popular works. I.Title.

Table of Contents

Avoiding and Surviving Breast Cancer

Prostate Cancer, BPH, & Better Sex for Men

Comments about Robert Bernardini's other books, *Everlasting Health* and *The Truth About Children's Health* *from PRI Publishing*

"This book is a masterpiece! A brilliant combination of modern science and innate wisdom, *Everlasting Health* is a compendium of invaluable information, resources, and references. Bernardini unravels the complexities, misunderstandings, and deceptions in our modern health-care system and serves up a compelling, original, and workable recipe for health. This book will save you money and can save your life and preserve life for our future generations."   Dale Paula Teplitz, M.A.

"This is the best health book I've ever read. I'm giving the extra copies I've ordered to friends and family – that's how important I think it is."   Donald L, Texas

"This is a vitally important book. The author has done his research and has discovered the probable causes for most illnesses and diseases. He then shows the courage to confront big business, the government, and the medical establishment, and reveals the misinformation that is propagated due to greed and power. He exposes the numerous dangers in our food supply and environment and then explains in clear and understandable English how to live to achieve optimal health. The fundamental theme throughout the book: We must live by the laws of nature in order to stay or become healthy. I think Robert's books are excellent!"   Tracy Cousins, M.D., Pathologist

"I used to spend about $200 a month on supplements. Since reading your book, last month I spent $0 and I feel better than ever!"   Stan J, Maryland

"...Your book is magnificent! It should be required reading in every school!"   W.E. Rose, California

"You are to be commended for all the years you have worked so hard to improve the health of mankind."   A.W. Thompson, Kentucky

"Robert's new book, *Everlasting Health*, is astonishingly comprehensive and really an encyclopedia of how to attain good health. I recommend you read it cover-to-cover with a highlighter and note pad handy. It concentrates on helping you address these problems in a supportive, holistic way, while at the same time shedding light on the oftentimes damaging effects of mainstream medical practices and drugs. Robert references an amazingly wide range of scientific research for validation which will allow any non-believer, that what's in this book is not hocus-pocus, but is indeed based on valid science. The most damaging thing you could do to your health might very well be to not read this book!"   David Getoff, CCN, CTN, CNC, FAAIM, Vice president of the non-profit Price-Pottenger Nutrition Foundation

"Bravo! Every Parent in America should have this book!"   Cheryl Peterson, massage therapist

Avoiding and Surviving Breast Cancer

Introduction

Breast cancer is the most common cancer among women in the U.S. with an estimated 240,510 new cases in 2007: Every 3 minutes a woman is diagnosed with breast cancer). It's the second leading cause of cancer deaths among women with 40,460 deaths in 2007, whereas there were 71,930 deaths from respiratory system cancers (lung, bronchus, and larynx). African American women are more likely to die of breast cancer than white women. Breast cancer incidence in women has increased from one in 20 in 1960 to one in eight today. It's not very well publicized, but men can get breast cancer too. An estimated 2,000 men will get breast cancer in 2007, and 450 of them will die from it. There are currently about 2 million breast cancer survivors in the U.S.[1,2]

As with many diseases, the medical community does not know what causes breast cancer. Risk factors of developing it include early puberty, late childbearing, obesity, use of oral contraceptives, no experience breast-feeding, heavy alcohol consumption and smoking. The biggest risk factor is age, since most breast cancers occur in women over the age of 50, and women over 60 are at the highest risk.[3]

The most common sign of breast cancer is a new lump or mass in the breast. A lump that is painless, hard, and has uneven edges means its likely cancer, but sometimes the lumps can be tender, soft, and rounded. Other signs include a swelling of part of the breast; skin irritation or dimpling; nipple pain or nipple turning inward; redness or scaliness of the nipple or breast skin; a clear, bloody, or yellow discharge from the nipple; and a lump in the underarm area. Cancerous breast lumps are firm and do not shrink and expand with the menstrual cycle. While most lumps are not cancerous, any breast abnormality should be brought to the attention of a doctor.

Clinical ways of detecting breast cancer include mammograms (an X-ray that detects abnormalities) and biopsy (a tissue sample is taken that is analyzed in a lab). A mammogram does not show whether you have cancer or not – it just shows overly dense tissue that may be cancerous. A biopsy is necessary to determine if the aberrant cells are cancerous. Denser breast tissue, as found in younger women, makes it harder to get an accurate mammogram. So for women under the age of 40 mammograms may not show much of anything.

There are five stages of breast cancer – 0 through IV – ranging from the cancer cells remaining inside the breast duct without invading normal breast

1

tissue, to the cancer spreading (metastasizing) to other parts of the body. Conventional treatments include surgery, radiation therapy, chemotherapy hormone therapy, and biological therapy. Oftentimes more than one of these therapies is used. The choice of treatment depends on the stage of the disease. Each of these treatments along with their hazards are presented below. Later on we will discuss alternative ways to address breast cancer, but for now, let's look at what a woman would be looking at if she addressed breast cancer in the conventional, mainstream way.

Food for Thought

You should always get a second opinion if diagnosed with cancer. The misdiagnosis rate for breast cancer is high – around 30 percent using mammograms. It's best to get a second opinion from a doctor in a different city, since doctors don't want to offend a colleague they know with a different diagnosis. Yes, this actually happens. You can call 1-800-4-CANCER for help with finding another doctor.

Getting breast cancer is very, very frightening. The 5 year survival rates range from 100 percent for Stage 0 and I, to just 20 percent for stage IV (Stage II – 92 percent; Stage III – 81 percent; Stage III – 54 percent)[4]

So if you get breast cancer, according to conventional medical statistics and using only conventional treatments, you have a pretty good chance of not being here 5 years after you're diagnosed. That's scary. It's so scary that most women do what the doctor says, even if it means having their breasts removed. It's hard to blame them. The mystique that doctors and the medical community have woven over the past 100 years has taken firm root in our minds. According to them, only they have the answers, only they have the cure.

Hopefully, you don't currently have breast cancer. If that's the case, you have a great opportunity to change the path you're on to ensure you'll never get it. If you do have breast cancer, changing your path is still a good idea. It may cause remission, or at least it will make the likelihood of recurrence less and recovery easier. If you have been diagnosed with breast cancer, consider this: It was reported in the *Archives of Surgery* that women who had undergone needle biopsies had a 50 percent greater risk of the cancer spreading to the lymph nodes, thereby reducing the subject's chance of survival. This suggests that disrupting a cancerous tumor with a needle may raise the risk of it spreading.[5] Just like with prostate cancer, it appears that leaving the tumor alone is better than sticking or cutting it.

Surgery for Breast Cancer

Surgical treatments for breast cancer can be divided into two classes: breast- sparing or mastectomy. Breast-sparing surgery includes a lumpectomy (removal of the malignant tumor only); segmental mastectomy; and partial mastectomy. Mastectomy surgery (where the whole of one or both breasts is removed) includes mastectomy (removal of the whole breast); a modified radical mastectomy (removal of breast and lymph nodes under the arm); and a radical mastectomy (removal of breast, lymph nodes and chest muscle).

Surgery is the most common treatment for breast cancer, and usually it's performed along with chemotherapy or radiation treatments before or afterwards. Obviously, losing part or all of a breast is a definite negative side effect along with any other side effects from surgery, chemo, or radiation. Many women who are told they could have breast-sparing surgery surprisingly opt to have a radical mastectomy anyway, thinking it will stop the chance that the cancer will reoccur or any cancer that was missed would spread.

Radiation Treatments

Radiation therapy uses high-energy rays of ionizing radiation to kill cancer cells (among other cells). Radiation therapy can be used before surgery to shrink the size of the tumor or after surgery to kill off any remaining cancer cells and (supposedly) stop any potential spread of cancer.

There are two types of radiation: external where the radiation comes from a large machine outside the body; and internal, where a radioactive substance is placed directly in the breast for several days. Side effects of radiation therapy include red, dry, tender, itchy, and weepy moist skin. Extreme fatigue is common and can last for a long time – sometimes years.

Chemotherapy Treatments

Chemotherapy uses anticancer drugs to kill cancer cells, administered as a pill or by injection so these drugs travel throughout the body. The side effects are vast and depend on the type of drug, amount taken and the length of treatment. Temporary side effects include fatigue, nausea, diarrhea, vomiting, loss of appetite, hair thinning and loss, being more prone to infections, and mouth sores. Changes in the menstrual cycle may be temporary or permanent, and low blood cell counts are typical.

Premature menopause and infertility (because the drugs damage the ovaries) are potential permanent complications and are more likely as a woman gets older. Rapid bone loss is a potential complication as is permanent heart damage. Getting pregnant while receiving chemotherapy could lead to birth defects.

Chemo brain may occur, meaning a decrease in mental function, concentration, and memory lasting up to a couple years after treatment. Rarely, one to two years after chemo, the drugs may cause acute myeloid leukemia – a life threatening cancer of the white blood cells. Generally, women who have received chemotherapy do not feel as healthy as they did before treatment, even years after the treatment has stopped. Fatigue is the biggest complaint.[6] There are some drugs that supposedly stop or lessen some of the side effects of chemotherapy.

Undoubtedly, chemotherapy is hazardous and uncomfortable. After all, its whole intent is to kill cells. Dr. William Campbell Douglass, an M.D. who considers alternative medical perspectives, has this to say about chemo and a possible alternative:

> Chemotherapy is the greatest crime committed by modern medicine. It is so illogical that I sometimes find it hard to believe that trained physicians from accredited universities subject cancer patients to its destructive effects. If the cancer is relatively benign, the chemotherapy will often "work" – despite the toxic nature of the treatment. But if it's benign, why put your body through chemotherapy when there are safer, nontoxic methods available that can produce even better results?[7]

Dr. Douglass goes on to tell of a man who was diagnosed with an aggressive form of non-Hodgkin's lymphoma, who conquered his cancer not by chemotherapy, but by changing his diet. This cancer survivor followed the nutritional principles of the Price-Pottenger Foundation or Weston A. Price Foundation, which are very similar to recommendations in the book *Everlasting Health* (see back cover).

Food for Thought

One overlooked hazard of getting cancer is that of developing a potentially fatal blood clot deep inside your leg. This is called deep vein thrombosis (DVT), and is the second leading cause of death among cancer patients. (A blood clot is a *thrombus*.) For people fighting some kinds of cancers, more than half died because of DVT. The risk of developing DVT for people taking chemotherapy drugs is twice as high as people free of cancer.

Complications from DVT blood clots kill around 200,000 people a year in the U.S., which is more than AIDS and breast cancer

4

combined. The classical symptoms of DVT include pain, swelling, and redness of the leg and dilatation of the surface veins. In up to 25 percent of all hospitalized patients, there may be some form of DVT, which often remains clinically unapparent

Typical treatment to prevent DVT is to administer anti-coagulation drugs like heparin or warfarin. But these also have their side effects. Following the recommendations for diet, exercise, rest, sleep, breathing and others found in the book *Everlasting Health* should keep you safe from blood clots, since your overall health, and thus the health of your blood, will be just fine. By the way, warfarin (trade name *Coumadin*) was originally used as a rat poison and is still in the same class of drugs (coumarins) as the contemporary rodenicides used today. They all interfere with blood coagulation by inhibiting vitamin K metabolism. Understandably, the side effects of warfarin are hemorrhaging (bleeding), coughing up blood, blood in the stools, bleeding from the nose and gums and even death.

Hormone Therapy

Hormone therapy or hormone treatment is used to add, block, or remove hormones in the body. Since certain hormones can attach to cancer cells and cause them to multiply, controlling the hormones might possibly control the cancer. The female hormones estrogen and progesterone can promote the growth of some breast cancer cells – so by blocking the production of these hormones, the cancer may not grow. (Hormone therapy for breast cancer is not the same as hormone replacement therapy, or HRT, used to treat the symptoms of menopause. More on that later.)

Hormone therapy consists of drugs (e.g., Tamoxifer, Fareston, Arimidex, Aromasin, Femara, Zoladex) to inhibit estrogen and progesterone. Sometimes surgery is used to remove the ovaries since they are the main supplier of estrogen. So a woman who has gone through menopause would not need that surgery since the ovaries produce less estrogen after menopause.

The drug most commonly used in hormone therapy is Tamoxifen (*Nolvadex*). It's a pill that's been used for breast cancer for 25 years, and is a type of drug called a selective estrogen-receptor modulator (SERM). It blocks estrogen from attaching to the estrogen receptors on cancer cells, and this prevents estrogen from exerting its growth stimulating effect on these cells thus conceivably halting the cancer.

The side effects of Tamoxifen are oftentimes similar to the symptoms of menopause – hot flashes and vaginal discharge. But other side effects include irregular menstrual periods, headaches, fatigue, nausea, vomiting, vaginal dryness and itching, irritation of the skin around the vagina, and skin rashes. More serious side effects are the formation of blood clots in the veins – most often in the legs and lungs. If one of these clots becomes loose, it could travel to the brain causing a stroke, or to the heart causing a heart attack.

Tamoxifen can cause cancer of the uterus, so it's recommended that women on this drug get regular pelvic exams and report any unusual activity such as bleeding in the vaginal area to their doctor. It's still possible to become pregnant while taking Tamoxifen (or any of the other drugs), and the drug may harm the fetus.

Biological Treatment

Biological therapy involves using a drug called Trastuzumab (*Herceptin*), a monoclonal antibody given intravenously that blocks a certain protein that slows or stops the growth of cancer. The side effects of this drug are fever, chills, weakness, nausea, vomiting, diarrhea, headaches, or rashes. In addition, it may cause heart damage that may lead to heart failure, and affect the lungs causing breathing problems. If that occurs, a doctor should be seen immediately. The benefits of this drug have been greatly manipulated to make it appear very helpful but the true statistical research show otherwise. Check out www.CancerDecisions.com

---

Food for Thought

Here's a question that most doctors and cancer treatment professionals wouldn't really appreciate, but needs to be asked: Why is it that even with surgery, chemo, radiation treatments, and the use of mammograms, the survival rates of breast cancer patients has not improved over the last 70 years?[8] With all the research going on and all the teases from the media about how science and technology is getting closer to a cure, why are just as many women dying of breast cancer as ever before?

Mammograms for Diagnosis of Breast Cancer

Mammograms are the most popular screening tool used by doctors. A mammogram involves firmly (and painfully) pressing your breast up against a plate and taking X-ray pictures of it from several angles. A survey in 2004 showed that nearly 90 percent of women who had no signs of the disease got screening mammograms, and most felt it would be irresponsible for a midlife woman not to.[9] Women are constantly admonished by the press, TV, medical establishment, and loved ones to get a mammogram "just to be

6

safe." After all, the American Medical Association, American Cancer Society and just about any doctor says a mammogram is the best way to catch breast cancer before it kills you.

True? Some other experts don't think so. Dr. Anthony Miller, Professor Emeritus at the University of Toronto, conducted a major study of mammography, studying 90,000 women in their 40s and 50s who had mammograms during breast exams or breast exams alone. He found that mammography helped detect more and smaller cancers, but did nothing to reduce death rates. In one part of the study, 105 of 25,214 women who had mammograms had died, and 107 of 25,216 women who had not had mammograms (just physical and self-exams) had died at the 13-year follow-up. This large sample and closely controlled study clearly shows no advantage to mammograms as far as death rate goes.(10,11,12)

Food for Thought

In response to learning that results of the study conduced by Dr. Miller mentioned above had been published in the *Journal of the National Cancer Institute*, Dr. Mercola, a well respected medical doctor, had this to say:

"Well now, here we have it: mammograms don't work. This is not published in some 'rinky-dink' journal or press release. This is from the National Cancer Institute. Their analysis confirms what we have suspected for some time that mammograms are not a good idea. Most physicians recommend them for fear of being sued by a woman who developed breast cancer after which he did not advise her to get one. Now natural medicine physicians can rest comfortably and encourage women to get a thorough breast examination for abnormalities, as well as perform frequent self-examinations."(13)

Allan Spreen, M.D. has another interesting comment:

"Back in my pathology residency, we examined cancerous breast tissue under the microscope. It was quite shocking to see, but many times I found a track of cancer cells extending out from the main tumor in a straight line. I came to find out this track of cancer cells was actually from a previous needle biopsy! Biopsies can actually disturb a tumor on a molecular level, pulling cancer cells into healthy breast tissue. I always felt a mammogram could do the same thing. A mammogram creates such intense pressure to the breast tissue (not to mention the radiation showered on the breast), it's possible that cancer cells could become dislodged."(14)

Another study published in the *Archives of Internal Medicine* in 2008 showed something even worse: mammograms actually increase breast cancer rates. Over 220,000 women were studied, and the women who had regular mammography screening (twice a year for six years) had a 22 percent higher rate of breast cancer than women who had but a single mammogram at the end of the six year period. The authors said, ". . .it appears that some breast cancers detected by repeated mammographic screening would not persist to be detectable by a single mammogram at the end of six years. This raises the possibility that the natural course of some screen-detected invasive breast cancers is to spontaneously regress." Meaning, the body can sometimes (and more than rarely) rid itself of cancer cells on its own.(15) Given half a chance, the body can do miraculous things. A Swedish study published in the *The Lancet* reported that the death rate from breast cancer among women under 55 was 29 percent higher in the group that had been screened with mammography compared to the unscreened control group. In addition, women in their 40s and 50s who had yearly mammograms actually had a 36 percent to 52 percent increase in breast cancer mortality.(16)

Mammograms aren't even reliable. In a Swedish study of 60,000 women, 70 percent of the tumors detected by mammography weren't tumors at all. Of the 5 percent of mammograms that suggested further testing, about 93 percent were false positives (showing cancer when there really was none).(17) Estimates are that 70 percent to 80 percent or all positive mammograms do not, upon biopsy, show any presence of cancer.

According to the National Cancer Institute, there is a high rate of missed tumors in women ages 40-49, resulting in 40 percent false negative test results (not showing cancer when there really was cancer). The National Institutes of Health admit that mammograms miss 25 percent of malignant tumors in women in their 40s, and 10 percent of malignant tumors in older women.(18,19,20)

Here's something else to think about: About one in four modern breast cancer diagnoses (using mammography) determine that the cancer is the slow developing ductal or lobular carcinomas (those that are in-situ – tumors still confined inside the ducts or lobules), which only become malignant, according to one report I read, about 2 percent of the time.(21) Another doctor said that between five and 20 percent of these kinds of cancers are malignant.(22) But oftentimes women are panicked into getting a mastectomy in these cases, when close monitoring would be sufficient. After all, only two out of 100 of these kinds of tumors become life threatening.(23) A thorough evaluation by you, your doctor, and a qualified oncologist is needed, and you need to get the real story on just what kind of tumor you have. Don't be afraid to ask questions and be demanding. It's your life.

Avoiding and Surviving Breast Cancer

Why might mammograms actually cause or worsen breast cancer? Two reasons: First, as Dr. Douglass says, "In what I call the 'compression syndrome,' the act of squeezing and compressing the breast in order to get good images during mammography may activate and spread an otherwise contained or localized mass of cancerous cells."[24] A tear in the tissue can cause a "leak" in the tumor, which allows the malignancy to spread and spread faster. In the old days, doctors were advised that breast lumps should be handled with care to prevent any such leak. Now? During a mammography, the breast is hardly handled with care. So in the same way that disturbing the prostate gland in a man might cause cancer cells to be activated, disturbing a woman's breast could activate the cancer too.

Second, the radiation used during a mammogram may cause the cancer. John W. Gofman, M.D, Ph.D., was a world renowned expert on radiation and Professor Emeritus in Molecular and Cell Biology at the University of California, Berkely. In his landmark book *Preventing Breast Cancer*, he states, "Our estimate is that about three-quarters of the current annual incidence of breast cancer in the United States is being caused by earlier ionizing radiation, primarily from medical sources."[25] His data show that the more mammograms a woman is subjected to, the greater her chances of getting breast cancer:

Age range	Number of Mammograms	Chance of Breast Cancer
30-34	1 exam	1 in 1,100
	5 exams	1 in 220
35-49	1 exam	1 in 1,900
	10 exams	1 in 190
50-64	1 exam	1 in 2,000
	15 exams	1 in 133

Dr. Gofman says that: radiation is a proven cause of human breast cancer; a woman's breast is more vulnerable to radiation than other parts of her body; breast irradiation during infancy and childhood increases the rate of breast cancer in adulthood; and, there is no safe dose of radiation – every exposure creates an increased rate of cancer in a population of cells.

A highly regarded group of health care analysts at the Cochrane Centre in Copenhagen, Denmark analyzed seven of the biggest and best studies on mammography screening. Their conclusion was that the best trials failed to show a significant reduction in breast cancer mortality. Even more, they said that because of mammographic screening, there are more breast cancer diagnoses and women of all ages undergo 31 percent more partial mastectomies, 20 percent more mastectomies and 24 percent more radiation treatments that do nothing to extend their lives.(26)

Dr. Gofman goes further, saying that medical radiation is a highly important cause, and probably the principal cause, of cancer mortality in the U.S. during the 20th Century. (Medical radiation includes X-rays, CT scans, and fluoroscopy.) He also says that medical radiation, even at very low and moderate doses, is an important cause of death from Ischemic Heart Disease due to it causing mini-tumors in the smooth muscles of the heart.

The Lancet reported that since mammographic screening was introduced in 1983, the incidence of ductal carcinoma in situ (DCIS) (which represents 12 percent of all breast cancer), has increased by 328 percent – 200 percent of this increase they conclude was due to the use of mammography.(27) These reports are compelling, to say the least, and hopefully will make you think twice before getting another X-ray, no matter where on your body or for what reason.

Alternatives to Mammograms

There are other tests that are being used as alternatives to mammograms. Two of them are good, two of them are not.

The AMAS (Anti-Malignant Antibody Screen) is a simple blood test that the originators claim can detect cancer cells of any type originating anywhere in the body. There is only one lab in the country doing the test (the people who say the test works) and the literature, testing and validation of this test is inconclusive and sketchy.

Then there's the new-fangled genetics testing that supposedly can reduce a woman's risk of developing cancer. However, these tests are not only expensive, but very limited and focused for certain genes such that it's estimated that perhaps just 1 percent of women without a family history of the disease would benefit from them.(28)

An alternative to mammograms that I do believe is effective, noninvasive and much safer is called thermography. This is not a blood test, but a way to detect possibly cancerous tissue by measuring infrared heat from the body. (A biopsy is necessary to determine if it's truly cancer.) It does not use any radiation.

One study showed that thermography had an over 95 percent predictive value and has revealed the presence of breast cancer despite normal reports from a mammogram (mammograms miss 10 percent of breast cancers).(29) Another study reported that thermography can detect 86 percent of non-palpable breast cancers and up to 15 percent of cancers that were not visible by mammography.(30) Thermography can detect a pathologic state of the breast up to 10 years before a cancerous tumor can be found by any other method, and has the ability to detect fast growing aggressive tumors.

The thermography test costs about $195 and some insurance companies cover the procedure. I think you'll see it become more and more popular as the years progress and people finally wake up to the fact that mammograms are not that good and can even be harmful. To find a doctor near you who uses thermography, or for more information, go to www.breastthermography.com. At the very least, if you think you must get mammograms, you could still get them, but less often, and use thermography to test the other times.

Another new test for breast cancer is Power Doppler Sonography (PDS) (also used to detect prostate cancer). It's very advanced ultrasound that can produce a detailed image (sonogram) of the body's internal structures and has a much higher resolution and the ability to highlight areas of blood flow in dense or soft tissue, allowing tumors or inflammation to be viewed and measured clearly. It can detect twice as many breast cancers as mammography and a study reported in the *British Journal of Urology* showed that this kind of test only misses 1 percent of prostate cancers.(31) Sonograms are safe, painless and inexpensive. Unlike other screening methods, they can be repeated as often as necessary to closely monitor areas of concern and assess treatment efficacy. For these reasons, sonograms have been found to be a more effective alternative to biopsies in detecting prostate tumors, and better than MRI and PET/CT scans as a means for tracking these tumors. PDS can also be used to monitor inflammation and tumors in the breast and other parts of the human body. To learn more and to find out where you can get one done, check out www.cancerscan.com and www.phoenixsonograms.com. Many health insurance companies are paying for these.

Food for Thought

Sonograms are also used in the detection of prostate cancer, Robert L. Bard, M.D., does these for both prostate and breast cancer. He is one of the world experts on cancer detection using this new, non-invasive, and incredibly accurate screening method. He says,

"About 25 percent of proven cancers will remain inactive in the breast and not grow or metastasize even in the absence of medical treatment. Many cancers are very low grade and grow slowly over 5-10 years before turning highly malignant. . .Some cancers grow rapidly and are highly malignant. These tumors seem to be best diagnosed by sonograms because sonography can detect a malignancy when it is ¼ inch in size and is highly accurate especially in high risk patients with

---

lumpy breasts where mammograms are of limited diagnostic value. . .The combined use of breast sonograms with Doppler blood flow study will provide early detection of most highly malignant cancers resulting in life saving early diagnosis and sparing the patient radical surgery. . .Sonography detects 4 times as many cancers as physical examinations and twice as many cancers as mammography."(32) Ladies, it's simple – instead of a mammogram, consider a sonogram.

Causes of Breast Cancer

Before we get into specifics, there's a comment by Peter Montague, editor of *Rachel's Environment & Health News* I want to share:

> The medical establishment dominated by male doctors pretends that the breast cancer epidemic will one day be reversed by some miracle cure, which we have now been promised for 50 years. Until that miracle arrives, we are told, there is nothing to be done except slice off women's breasts, pump their bodies full of toxic chemicals to kill cancer cells, burn them with radiation, and bury our dead. Meanwhile, the normal public health approach of primary prevention languishes without mention and without funding. We know what causes the vast majority of cancers: exposure to carcinogens. What would a normal public health approach entail? Reduce the burden of cancer by reducing our exposure to carcinogens. One key idea has defined public health for more than 100 years: PREVENTION.(33)

Although the medical establishment insists they don't know the cause of breast cancer (so they can continue to get funding for their drug research), it is fairly obvious if you review the scientific literature: Most breast cancers are caused by exposure to chemicals, endocrine-disrupting chemicals, drugs, and ionizing radiation. Other causes could include deficiencies in selenium and iodine as well as over consumption of sugars and processed starches.

Chemicals

A Japanese women living in Japan has about one quarter the risk of getting breast cancer has her American counterpart. When Japanese women move to America, by the second generation, their risk of breast cancer has risen to "normal" American levels. We must conclude that something in the environment and diet, not genetics, is at work here.

Avoiding and Surviving Breast Cancer

In Israel, deaths from breast cancer in young women less than 44 years old in the 1960s and 1970s began to sharply increase. Then, the death rate from breast cancer in women 44 or younger dropped between 1976 and 1989: but the death rate among older Israeli women continued to rise. That was an unusual pattern. Was there an explanation?

There was. In the 1970s, measurements of three carcinogenic pesticides in cow's milk and human milk in Israel found levels five to 1,000 times higher than in the U.S. These contaminants were Lindane (since banned in U.S.), DDE (a chemical created when DDT breaks down in the environment) and alpha-BHC. Cow's milk and human tissues were all found to be heavily contaminated with these. Finally, in 1978, after public protests, Israel banned these pesticides. By 1980, breast milk contamination had dropped 90 percent or more among the Israeli women.(34)

Could these pesticides have caused the unusual breast cancer pattern in Israel? Many scientists think so. A recent study in America showed women with breast cancer have significantly elevated levels of DDT, DDE, and PCBs in their fat compared to women who do not have cancer.(35) The incidence of breast cancer goes down when a woman exercises on a regular basis, and eats more green vegetables and fiber.

Food for Thought

The connection between breast milk and toxicity is not intended to discourage you from breastfeeding your baby. Breast feeding gives an infant immunity against gastrointestinal diseases and respiratory infections, offers protection against food allergies, provides emotional bonding between mother and child, and is really the right food for the baby. Prepared formulas and baby foods are usually even more contaminated than mother's milk.

Human breast milk can also be affected by pollution. Scientists first discovered human breast milk was contaminated with DDT in 1951. DDT, like many other chlorinated organic chemicals (pesticides), is soluble in fat but not very soluble in water. So when it enters the body, it's not easily excreted and builds up in fatty tissue. Breast milk contains about 3 percent fat and fat-soluble chemicals collect there. So, if the mother is contaminated and she breastfeeds her baby, the baby gets contaminated too.

In 1975 the EPA conducted a study of the milk of American women. Taking samples from more than one thousand women and analyzing them for only a few pesticides, they found DDT in 100 percent of the samples, PCBs in 99 percent, and dieldrin in 83 percent. All three are considered probable carcinogens by the EPA.(36)

Until early 1999, pesticides had never been measured in the amniotic fluid of pregnant women. (The amniotic fluid is what the fetus floats in the womb prior to birth.) But in June 1999, researchers in the United States and Canada found p,p'-DDE (a breakdown byproduct of DDT), in 30 percent of the women examined. The concentrations of p,p'-DDE found in the amniotic fluid are a real concern. Of the various health problems associated with these chemicals, developmental abnormalities of the male reproductive tract, suppression of immune function, development of the brain, and neurobehavioral problems in children are of major concern because they are irreversible. DDE is known to interfere with male sexual development by deactivating the male sex hormone, testosterone.(37)

Endocrine-disrupting Chemicals

Hormones and growth factors act as chemical messengers in the body and are important in the normal growth and functioning of cells and tissues, including breast tissue. However, they can also play a role in the development of cancer, especially when they come from external and unnatural sources.

There is much evidence that links breast cancer to "xenoestrogens," chemicals strange or foreign to the human body that mimic or interfere with the body's natural estrogen, the female sex hormone. Indeed, many common industrial chemicals and pesticides mimic these hormones and thus interfere with fundamental bodily processes. DDT, methoxychlor, benzene, and others can act like sex hormones and interfere with fundamental biological processes such as reproduction in wildlife and humans. It is believed that xenoestrogens stimulate the growth of cells in the breast, possibly giving rise to cancer.(38)

From epidemiological studies (studies of diseases in the human population), there's evidence that exposure of females to xenoestrogens while in the womb can increase their risk of breast cancer as adults. Not only that, but if a male is exposed to these same chemicals while in the womb, it reduces his ability to produce sperm later in life. It's estimated that the average male today produces only half as much sperm as his grandfather did, and exposure to environmental toxins may well be the cause of this decline. (If this decline were to continue at historical rates, humans in industrialized countries would have difficulty reproducing themselves by about the year 2020.) There is also evidence that prostate cancer, the second leading cause of cancer deaths in the U.S. for men, (lung cancer is number one), is linked to these xenoestrogens.(39)

14

There are probably hundreds of substances that mimic naturally occurring hormones from pesticides, cleansers, solvents, plasticizers, surfactants, dyes, cosmetics, PCBs, and dioxins.

Hormone Replacement Therapy

Hormone Replacement Therapy (HRT) is designed to ease the transition through menopause and lessen symptoms such as hot flashes, vaginal dryness, mood swings, sleep disorders and decreased sexual desire. Drugs for this use include the hormones estrogen and progesterone (usually synthetic progestin), which are usually administered by pill, patch, or vaginal cream. The most popular brand name is *Prempro*. Estrogen is oftentimes used alone, the most popular brand name being *Premarin*.

A large-scale study on the combination drug using estrogen and progesterone (*Prempro*) was started in 1993 by the National Institutes of Health (NIH). By 2002, the study was halted three years early because so many women were having serious health problems, most notably, an increased rate of breast cancer.

The results of the study showed that women taking these drugs experienced: 26 percent increase in breast cancer; 41 percent increase in strokes; 29 percent increase in heart attacks; twice as many blood clots; and; 22 percent increase in total cardiovascular disease.[40] Other health problems in study participants included coughing up blood, vision problems, nausea, hair loss, headaches, depression, decreased libido, weight gain and fatigue.[41]

Food for Thought

Since 1942 when these drugs were introduced, the estrogen in *Prempro* and *Premarin* has come from the urine of pregnant mares (female horses). To get the urine, the mares are forced to stand in stalls less than five feet wide 24/7 with urine collection devices strapped to them. They are unable to turn, lie down or exercise, and the devices strapped to them can cause infections and chafing. In the last months of their eleven-month pregnancy, the mares are put out to pasture to have their foals (baby horses). Then, they're put in a herd with a stallion so they become pregnant again as soon as possible, and their foals are taken away from them even if they're not fully weaned. Once pregnant again, it's back into the pee barn so more urine can be collected.

Besides the cruel treatment of the mares, the foals are oftentimes slaughtered and their meat shipped to Europe and Japan. When the mare can no longer get pregnant, she is slaughtered too. All told, it's

---

estimated that over the years, the production of these drugs has cost the lives of over a million horses.(42) Besides these drugs being bad for the women who take them, realize that every time they're prescribed, untold misery is inflicted on those poor horses.

But will that stop the manufacturer, Wyeth, from promoting these products? Hardly. After all, they make about $1 billon a year from the sales of *Premarin, Prempro,* and two other drugs along the same line, *Premphase* and *Prempac.* In fact, Wyeth has successfully lobbied the FDA to ban (January 9, 2008) the use of the natural hormone estriol in estrogen medications. Estriol, a *bioidentical hormone,* has been used successfully for years without major health problems. But when Wyeth's profits dropped more than 57 percent ($2.07 billion in 2003 to $800 million in 2004) after the above mentioned study was released showing serious side effects of these drugs, they had to do something!

Concerning treatment for menopausal symptoms, Dr. Mercola says, "If you are going to use hormone replacement therapy, clearly bioidentical hormones are the way to go and an absolute no-brainer if one has had a surgically induced menopause."(43)
Bioidentical hormones are those that are made to be the same as the hormone your body would have produced. This is as opposed to using a synthetic or horse hormone.

It's estimated that in 2002, 22 million women were taking *Premarin* for menopausal symptoms. But when the study mentioned above was released that year showing the link between HRT and all those other health problems, not surprisingly, many women stopped taking it. This study funded by the National Institute of Health as part of the Women's Health Initiative was cut short because of the higher incidences of health problems the participants were having.)(44)

What happened? Breast cancer rates in America declined by 7.2 percent the year after the study was published (14,000 fewer women were diagnosed with the disease in 2003). The symptoms of menopausal may include hot flashes, vaginal dryness, mood swings, sleep disorders and decreased sex drive – all discomforts to be sure, but usually not life threatening (as are the problems with the drugs).

About 30 percent of American women over the age of 50 have taken HRT between 2000 and 2005. That's a lot of women.(45) The study was conducted on 161,809 women ages 50-79, from 40 different medical centers – a pretty good size study. Once again, a drug is shown to cause more problems than it fixes.

Food for Thought

Hormones are big business. It all started back in 1934 when American drug companies began selling synthetic hormones to be used in cosmetics, drugs, food additives, and animal feed. The best known of these hormones is diethylstilbestrol (DES). It didn't take long to realize it could cause cancer: In 1938 and again in 1941, studies were reported by the National Cancer Institute that showed DES caused breast cancer in rodents. But DES is 400 times as potent as natural estrogen and can be made very cheaply, so instead of banning its use because it caused breast cancer in women, the FDA, bless their hearts, approved its use in 1941.

Since then, DES has been used as a morning after pill to prevent pregnancy, to prevent miscarriages, and as a breast-enlarging cream. As early as 1947, adverse effects of DES were reported among U.S. women who ate chicken treated with this hormone. In 1971, human cancer from DES was confirmed, and it was banned from meat in 1973. But other growth hormones are now used instead to fatten animals. These hormones are used to promote cell and tissue growth, and cause weight gain. (You wonder why so many people are fat? The hormones end up in *us*.) So is it really surprising that they would also promote cancer cell growth? Not everyone thinks that hormones are good – Europe will not allow U.S. meat be imported because of the U.S.'s ubiquitous use of hormones in animal feed.(46)

Concerning chemicals, Europe has eliminated 900 compounds for use in beauty products due to their suspected role in causing cancer, genetic mutations, and reproductive disorders. They banned the use of phthalates (a chemical used in plastics and resins) in nail polish in 2004. Europe has also restricted the use of six phthalate compounds in toys. Although manufacturers in the U.S. said they would limit their use in toys voluntarily, they are still being used today.(47)

Common characteristics shared by many women who end up developing breast cancer include: early menarche; late menopause; late childbirth and no children or the birth of few; lack of breast-feeding; obesity; a high fat diet; being tall; taking oral contraceptives; cancer of the ovaries or uterus; and excessive use of alcohol.

"What is the message running through all of these risk?" ask Dr. Janet Sherman, author of *Life's Delicate Balance – The Causes and Prevention of Breast Cancer*. "Hormone, hormones, and hormones. Hormones of the wrong kind, hormones too soon in a girls' life, hormones for too many years in a woman's life, too many chemicals with hormonal action, and too great a total hormonal load."[48]

Excess Weight

Weight gain during adult life, especially after menopause, increases the risk of breast cancer, and weight loss after menopause decreases the risk of getting it. There's between a 4 percent and 24 percent higher risk of breast cancer for women who have gained at least 2 kg of weight since age 18. Researchers said ". . .we estimated that 15 percent of post-menopausal breast cancer cases in our population may be attributable to weight gain of 2.0 kg [4½ lbs] or more since age 18 years and 4.4 percent attributable to weight gain of 2.0 kg or more since menopause."[49]

Deodorants and Cosmetics

Of special concern are findings that makeup and underarm deodorants and antiperspirants can increase the risk of developing breast cancer. Both products often contain parabens (a preservative found in lotions, shampoo, sunscreen, skin foundation, bath gels and deodorants), that has been shown to act like a weak estrogen. Parabens have been found with regularity in breast tumors, and are thought to have estrogenic effects in estrogen-sensitive human cells (which breast cells are). Notably, 60 percent of all breast tumors are located in the upper-outer quadrant, nearest the underarm where deodorants are typically applied.[50]

One researcher, Dr. Kris McGrath, showed that women who shaved at least three times a week and applied antiperspirants at least twice a week were almost 15 years younger when diagnosed with cancer than women who did neither. Dr. McGrath believes that's it's the aluminum in the antiperspirant that is the culprit. Usually they don't penetrate the skin, but when the skin is freshly shaven, they do.[51]

Food for Thought

For a natural deodorant, take a lemon wedge and rub under the arms. Adding a little ginger helps too. If you must use store-bought antiperspirants, please get one that doesn't contain aluminum, since it is believed to contribute to Alzheimer's disease. Since sweating is one of the body's main methods of detoxification, and since the breast is immediately adjacent to the underarms, it may be that reducing the detoxification (sweating) in this area could easily increase breast cancer. Use a nontoxic *deodorant* and NOT an *anti-perspirant*.

Cosmetics are typically not only laden with parabens, but contain phthalates too. These chemicals have been linked to certain birth defects and also can disrupt the natural hormones balance in the body, which may in turn increase the risk of breast cancer.

Not only that, but a study by Dr. Janet Gray at Vassar College suggests that women who begin using makeup at an earlier age and in greater amounts may have an increased risk of developing breast cancer later in life. It appears that shampoos and other hair care products, especially those marketed to the African-American community, are the worst offenders. These products have extracts from placentas (to strengthen hair and reduce breakage), which contain adult hormones like estrogen.(52)

Dr. Gray says, "Adolescence is the time when breasts are developing, so this is clearly a time when exposure matters for developing breast cancer 20 to 30 years later." For a list of cosmetic product that are supposed to be free of these chemicals, go to www.safecosmetics.org.

Antibiotics, Aspirin, Antidepressants and Smoking

A study reported in the *Journal of the American Medical Association* states that antibiotic use is associated with an increased risk of breast cancer, and the more antibiotics used, the more the risk increased. The study of over 10,000 women found that those who took antibiotics for more than 500 days (or had more than 25 prescriptions for the drugs over a period of 17 years or so) had more than twice the likelihood of developing breast cancer compared to women who didn't use any antibiotics.(53) Even if a woman had between one and 25 prescriptions over the same period, they are one-and-a-half times more likely to get it. Researchers aren't sure why, but the evidence is compelling.

Food for Thought

It's not surprising that antibiotics use can lead to cancer, be it breast or any other kind. Antibiotics kill (they are poisons, after all) bacteria which, believe it or not, help to keep our bodies clean of metabolic wastes and toxins from the outside world. See more in the book *Everlasting Health.*

A study of 114,000 women in California showed some alarming trends in those who took aspirin and/or ibuprofen and the development of breast cancer. The daily use of aspirin for five years or more caused a dramatic increase in breast cancer, and those taking ibuprofen every day for at least five years increased a woman's chances of developing breast cancer by 50 percent compared to those who did not use the drugs regularly.(54)

How about antidepressants? Women taking paroxetine (*Paxil*) were shown to have a seven-fold increased risk of breast cancer in one study.(55) Women taking tricyclic antidepressants (TCAs) were found to have about twice the risk of developing the disease.(56) These findings have been known since 2000, but has the general public, or even the doctors prescribing these medicines, heard about them?

Smoking, not surprisingly, can increase the risk of developing breast cancer too. Women who were current smokers had about a 30 percent greater chance of getting this cancer than those who had never smoked. But, the good news is, there's no evidence of significantly increased breast cancer risk among women who had previously smoked but had quit.(57)

Bras

A husband and wife team of medical anthropologists has done intriguing research they say indicates that wearing a bra can cause breast cancer and fibrocystic breast disease. Sydney Ross Singer and Soma Grismaijer surveyed 4,730 women to determine their bra-wearing habits and incidences of diseases. They found that women who wore their bras 24 hours a day had a three out of four chance of developing breast cancer. Women who wore bras more than 12 hours a day had a one in seven chance. Those who wore one less than 12 hours a day had a one in 152 risk, and women who wear bras rarely or never had a one in 168 chance of getting breast cancer.

Although this study was not a scientifically controlled study, the results are compelling. Singer and Grismaijer believe the pattern is due to the constricting nature of the bra, which hinders or stops lymph flow. Lymph is the garbage-disposal system of the body, and is totally dependant on movement since there's no pump for it. If the breast and surrounding tissues are bound tight, they're not able to receive the gentle massage during everyday movements and walking that move the lymph and help cleanse the tissues. The lymph fluid accumulates in the breast tissue and this accumulation leads to breast tenderness, pain, and ultimately the fluid turns into cysts.

There are reports that within days or weeks of stopping wearing a bra, the breast tissue is allowed to flush out the excess fluid, the cysts disappear and the breast pain and tenderness go away. Singer and Grismaijer say that getting rid of the bra has resulted in over 95 percent recovery of pain and cyst problems.(58) Therefore, it's probably best not to sleep in a bra, and perhaps wear one less during the day if possible. Singer and Grismaijer wrote a book that discusses this in detail titled *Dressed to Kill*, that you can find on the internet.

Most bras are made of fabric that contains petrochemicals. Having that next to your skin for hours on end can't be good. When you do wear a bra, try to have it be of natural fibers.

Food for Thought

Not surprisingly, the American Cancer Society (ACS) debunked Singer and Grismaijer's research because it ". . .was not conducted according to standard principles of epidemiological research and did not take into consideration other variables, including known risk factors for breast cancer."(59) OK, maybe it wasn't the perfect study. (Which one is?) But the research at least points to a possible contributing factor for breast cancer. So with such compelling evidence, why doesn't the ACS design and conduct a study that meets their criteria so we can see if maybe something as simple as wearing a bra less than 12 hours per day could make a difference? Simple: It won't make them money.

I'm not sure if it's just human nature or the "powers that be"' are intentionally twisting things so the innocent and trustworthy keep following their dogma, but the end result is us spending money in directions that have in the past, not proven fruitful. How many times do we hear: "We're getting closer to a cure. We need to do more research to find out. It may be a virus, it may be genetics, we just don't know. We need more money to do the research to find out. Please give to _____."

So millions of well intentioned Americans give millions of dollars a year to the cancer foundations, heart foundations, diabetes foundations and countless others. There are walkathons and pink ribbons and teddy bears for sale with funds going to medical research. And what does this research do? Aside from a few token studies on nutrition and environmental factors, the overwhelming bulk of the money for research goes into answering one question: "what drug can we invent, patent and sell to treat it?"

But there are problems with that. First, drugs don't heal. They simply can't – only the body can heal and the body can only heal when it is supplied with the proper nutrients to do so. Drugs just alter and alleviate symptoms (at the expense of the overall health of the body since they are toxins the body must handle). Second, drug companies and researchers make their living from sick people. Why should they find a cure when they make so much money chasing one? So they'll say they're making advances, and things are better than they used to be and the cure is just around the corner. It's not. The health of Americans is getting worse and worse. (Partly because of all the drugs we're consuming. Drug residues are even now in our water supplies.) With all the billions and billions of dollars spent over the years on research to find "the cure", why do survival rates remain essentially unchanged?

This "we-need-drugs" mindset has to change. There are TV drug commercials for prostate problems, depression, impotence, osteoporosis, cholesterol, heart conditions, colds, flu, heart-burn, allergies, bi-polar disorder, bladder weakness, cervical cancer, even restless legs. Someone made the observation that this generation of kids who are exposed to this drug media blitz, will, by the time they are adults, think it's perfectly natural to have these diseases and that the only way to treat them is with drugs. All this advertising is not just to sell drugs now, but to brainwash all the children and teens into believing that taking them is as normal a way of life as washing your hair. (Have you noticed all the cartoon characters like butterflies or cute bumblebees in the ads? Just like Joe Camel smoking cigarettes years ago before he was banned because his cartoon nature influenced children.)

When you think drugs, think unnatural chemicals – which is what all drugs are. Chemicals do nothing to nourish, nurture, or heal the body and are all poisonous to one degree or another. Drugs simply mask symptoms which reappear in another form later on. For true healing, or to reverse cancer, heart disease or any other malady, we must do two things. One, stop doing the things that are causing the disease in the first place. This amounts to eliminating from our environment and food supply toxins which damage cells and cellular processes. Two, nourish and care for the body so that nature can use its wisdom to heal us. If we supply the body the tools, mother nature will do her job. Few people realize this these days. Most believe only drugs and technology can heal. We have lost sight of the truth, due in large part to the advertising and fear the drug companies use to convince us we need them.

So next time you see a rally for breast cancer or diabetes research or the heart fund, think again. You may want to spend your money on clean and nutritious food instead of giving it away to researchers who are just chasing their tails. I know this may sound hard and insensitive, but it is not. Technology or drugs are not smarter or more effective than nature, and you're just supporting and encouraging a fundamentally flawed (and greedy) system that makes plenty of promises with no progress. If you want to make a donation, give to foundations who promote healthy living and proper nutrition. Two of them are: The Price-Pottenger Nutrition Foundation (www.ppnf.org); and, The Weston A. Price Foundation (www.westonaprice.org).

Around election time, you'll always hear a politician say something like, "I'll make sure that all Americans, especially the elderly, can get the drugs they need!" Like he's doing us a *favor*? Like that's one of our unalienable rights? Some day, some brave soul will get up and say something like,

"My dear Americans. We need to rebuild America from the ground up. If elected, I will make sure that our farmlands are replenished with all the minerals they need to grow healthy and nutritious crops; for as Pulitzer Prize winning author and agriculturist Louis Bromfield said, ". . . one of the great problems of American agriculture [is] the decline of human stock through the decline in fertility and mineral content of the soil itself. *'Poor land makes poor people'* is a saying every American should have printed and hung over his bed."(60) I will ensure that every one of us, young and old alike, can get inexpensive organically raised food, meat without hormones, eggs from free-range hens, raw milk and wholesome cod liver oil a-plenty. I'll get the additives, artificial sweeteners, and preservatives out of our food supply and make sure that we, and especially our children, are not forced into being shot up with poisons. I'll make it possible for you to have the time to get adequate sunshine and plenty of exercise. If I'm elected, I pledge to you to take all the money that goes into drug research and development and spend it on cleaning up our food supply and the environment and making sure all products are non-toxic. My fellow Americans, deep down in your hearts, you know. . .you *know*. . . that only nature can heal and it is our unalienable right to be given the opportunity to simply allow it to do so. We've been deceived by the greedy and power-hungry for too long! It's time for a change – a REAL change, literally from the ground up! It's time to rise up and say no more! No more deception! No more lies! No more weakening of the American body and spirit just to make a buck! If you are strong enough, brave enough, resilient enough and insightful enough, you'll see that the natural way is the only way to true health and happiness. Yes, if you're brave enough, you can rise above the pain and suffering. You can rise up and ensure that your children and future generations will be able to claim our God-given right – our right to natural and everlasting health! Then, and only then, will America be restored to greatness!" That would be quite a speech, don't you think?

As an environmental engineer, I had the opportunity to inspect many factories and manufacturing plants. The factories and kinds of facilities I saw ran the gamut from metal plating operations, textile mills, and nuclear power plants all the way to chicken processing plants, car washes, and Laundromats. I saw quite an assortment of nasty and dirty problems, since my job was to make sure the facilities were kept clean and their wastes were disposed of properly.

One day while in the office, a number of inspectors were comparing notes, and the question was raised which kind of facility we disliked inspecting most. The answer was unanimous – pharmaceutical plants. They were the nastiest, dirtiest, stinkiest, most toxic places we saw, and that's saying something. The one I had to inspect regularly had hoses and cans strewn about, puddles of chemicals, pipes leaking slime. At the end of the employee's parking lot, there were several sprayers that hosed your car off as you left. I asked the vice-president why it was there, and he said that if you didn't hose your car off at least a couple times a week, it would start to corrode and just melt away because the air around the plant was so caustic. One of the VP's walked with a limp, one had an incessant eye twitch, and there was the story of the man who worked there whose skin turned bright orange (I never met the man, he died before I started going there). There were massive fish kills in the river downstream of the plant and trees around the plant died. We forced them to build berms to control run-off, spend millions to improve their wastewater treatment plant, and do groundwater reclamation. That's not to mention all the air quality control things another department forced them to do. All in all, it was a very toxic and dangerous place. And what did they make there? Heart medicine and anti-inflammatory drugs.

Seeing what really goes on at pharmaceutical plants and just how drugs are made and what is used to make them made a big impression on me: I haven't taken any kind of drug, pill, potion, or medicine of any kind since then. That was over 20 years ago. It was like pulling the curtain away from the Wizard of Oz – just an imposter with a lot of hot air.

Avoiding Breast Cancer

Sunlight and Vitamin D

People who live in warm and sunny climates have less risk of developing some cancers, and it's been documented that people in northeastern states have a higher mortality rate from breast, colon and other types of cancer than people living in southern states. The death rate is directly related to the amount of solar radiation received, and the closer you get to the equator, the lower your risk of breast-cancer death.(61,62,63) Now researchers are trying to determine just how much vitamin D is needed for breast cancer prevention. Cedric Garland, DPH of the University of California San Diego suggested in the American Association for Cancer Research annual meeting in 2006 that increasing intake of vitamin D can lower the chance of developing breast cancer by 10 percent to 50 percent.(64)

The average vitamin D intake in the U.S. is 320 IU/day, which is only about one tenth the amount to be associated with a 50 percent reduction of breast cancer incidence. "We believe that higher doses of vitamin D will product proportionate reductions in the incidence of breast cancer. . .It's nearly impossible to get enough vitamin D in your diet alone," Garland says. An 8-ounce glass of milk contains only 100 IU of vitamin D and a serving of cereal has 20 IU. He recommends taking 1,000 IU of vitamin D (in the form of D_3, not D_2), especially during the winter months. By comparison, someone who spends 10 to 15 minutes in the sun on a sunny day without sunscreen can absorb 2,000 to 5,000 IU of vitamin D if 40 percent of the body is exposed. (65,66)

Researchers in Canada have also shown vitamin D to be important in breast cancer prevention, and found that exposure to sunshine early in life (especially between the ages of 10 to 19) had a significant effect on whether a woman gets breast cancer later in life. "Current thinking is that exposures during adolescence or before a full-term pregnancy may have a greater effect, as that is when breast tissue is going through the most rapid development," Dr. Knight says. In addition, taking vitamin D-rich cod liver oil between ages 10 and 19 reduced breast cancer risk by about 35 percent later in life.(67)

Magnesium

Magnesium is critical for the proper function of the endocrine system, which makes and balances the hormones that play such an important role in breast cancer genesis. Specifically, if the body does not receive enough magnesium, the delicate balance of hormones will suffer. And since about 75 percent of all breast cancers are stimulated by estrogen, it's important that it be maintained at its proper level.

Magnesium is necessary for the production of cholesterol, from which all the sex hormones (estrogen, testosterone) as well as aldosterone and DHEA (dehydroepiandrosterone) are made (another reason you need cholesterol). It's vital for the proper function of the pituitary gland (the *master gland*), which helps balance hormones, and the pineal gland, which helps regulate sleep. Since an overabundance of estrogen is a primary cause of breast cancer, it's important to keep all the hormones in balance.

Since magnesium is instrumental in the regulation of hormones, it not only plays a role in breast cancer, but is also important during menopause. During menopause, the natural secretion of estrogen is decreased, and signs of aging and discomfort are common. Dr. Norman Shealy, an expert on anti-aging, says he has found that through the transdermal (across the skin) use of magnesium, women have reported complete abatement of menopausal symptoms and some have even returned to their menstrual cycle.[68]

This improvement did not occur when magnesium was taken orally, but by spreading a product called *magnesium oil* on the skin and letting it soak in. It's been reported that serum magnesium levels can be raised higher and faster using this product since it doesn't cause diarrhea as large oral doses of magnesium does. In addition, magnesium oil contains magnesium chloride, the form of magnesium the body assimilates most readily.

Dr. Melvyn R. Werbach believes that borderline magnesium levels seen in premenstrual syndrome (PMS) can explain most of the symptoms associated with it. Double-blind studies have shown that magnesium supplementation has relieved these symptoms. Dr Werbach says that a marginal deficiency of magnesium can deplete levels of dopamine, impair estrogen metabolism, increase insulin secreting and cause the enlargement of the adrenal cortex, which produces many hormones including sex hormones, stress hormones and blood-sugar hormones.[69]

It's estimated that up to 80 percent of American women experience hot flashes or other symptoms of menopause vs. just 10 percent of Japanese women. It's thought that this is probably due to the fact that the Japanese eat so much seaweed, which is very high in magnesium.

Since a magnesium deficiency can cause blood vessels to go into spasm thus causing a menstrual migraine, additional magnesium can help delay or eliminate these headaches. Magnesium taken orally during the last 15 days of the menstrual cycle has been shown to sometimes prevent these types of migraines.[70] Of course, each woman's body is different and has different needs, so there's no guarantee just taking a few magnesium pills will prevent a headache. Based on the research, using the magnesium oil is much more effective than oral supplementation. In fact, Dr. Sircus says that only one-third to one-half of dietary magnesium is absorbed into the body, and we need about 1,000 mgs a day just to keep up with daily demands. So he highly recommends using the magnesium oil to obtain this kind of intake.

Eating a diet high in magnesium (drinking fresh vegetable juices) and avoiding things that rob your body of magnesium (alcohol and all drugs) is still the best way to go. All in all, magnesium is a great mood enhancer, muscle relaxant and even helps in temperature regulation (helps those hot flashes). So it may be helpful to give nature's tranquillizer a try.

Iodine

Animals in an iodine deficient state are more likely to develop breast cancer, and the longer the diet is deficient in iodine, the more likely it will develop.[71,72,73] An iodine deficiency also encourages breast tissue to respond more to estrogen, which, we know, will increase the likelihood of cancer.[74]

Unfortunately, the American diet is lacking in iodine, and the recommended daily allowance (RDA: 150 mcg/day for adult male to 290 mcg/d for lactating woman), many experts now believe is too low. Dr. David Brownstein, a leading proponent of iodine, says, "Iodine deficiency, coupled with exogenous estrogens from the diet (e.g. hormones fed to animals) or chemicals in the environment (e.g., phthalates from plastics), could explain the epidemic of breast cancer that is occurring in this country (as well as in many other western countries)."[75]

The Japanese eat a large amount of seaweed, which is rich in magnesium. Seaweed is also one of the best sources of iodine, allowing the Japanese to consume about 13.8 mg of iodine per day. This is 100 times more than the U.S. RDA for iodine. Japanese women have remarkably lower levels of breast cancer (and endometrial and ovarian cancers as well). Further, when Japanese women move to the U.S., their rates of mortality from breast, endometrial and ovarian cancer increases. Other studies show that countries with higher intakes of iodine have lower rates of breast cancer (and goiter); and countries with lower intakes of iodine have higher incidences of breast cancer (and goiter).[76]

In contrast, the average daily intake of iodine in the U.S. is just 240 micrograms (or 0.24 mg) of iodine, which is less than 2 percent of what the Japanese consume.[77] Dr Donald W. Miller, Jr., noted that about 15 percent (one in seven) women in the U.S. probably suffers from iodine deficiency and one in seven American women now develop breast cancer. Thirty years ago, only one in twenty women developed breast cancer, and the consumption of iodine was significantly greater.

These observations are consistent with medical research. Studies show that high intake of iodine is associated with low incidence of breast cancer, and low intake of iodine is associated with high incidence of breast cancer.[78,79]

Is there a connection between iodine consumption and breast cancer? Many experts now believe so. But it's not like this link is anything new: The relationship between low iodine levels and breast cancer was noted in modern medical journals as early as 1960, and the first time iodine was used to treat breast cancer was in 1896.[80,81]

Breast tissue is one of the body's main storage and utilization sites for iodine. But since the thyroid gland is the organ that uses and needs iodine the most, when the diet is deficient in iodine, the thyroid gets it first, and the breast tissue (and other tissues) has to wait. Since iodine is so important to proper functioning of breast tissue, a supply that more than meets the needs of the thyroid gland is needed. How much is this? Brownstein says adults should consume between 6 mg and 50 mg of iodine per day.

Besides cancer, iodine is important in another disease of the breast, which may turn into cancer – that being fibrocystic breast disease. This disease has increased from 3 percent in the 1920s to 90 percent of women today. The symptoms include fluid-filled cysts, fibrosis with tenderness and breast pain that lasts more than six days during the menstrual cycle. In short, there are lumps that are hard and painful.

Russian researchers reported that 71 percent of women who had the disease were healed by taking 50 mg per day of potassium iodide (KI). Other studies in America found similar findings (70 percent success rate) when iodine was given in therapeutic amounts.[82,83,84]

Dr. Brownstein also reports that iodine is extremely effective in treating and preventing fibrocystic breasts, and that iodine has been the most researched mineral in treating this disease. He says that after iodine supplementation is started, women typically see a rapid improvement with the cysts and pain disappearing within a few months. If there's no improvement by then, then the disease is probably caused by other factors.[85]

Guy Abraham, M.D., Jorge Flechas, M.D., and David Brownstein, M.D. started what they called the Iodine Project in 2003 to study the effects of higher than normal consumptions of iodine. In this study, volunteers took 12.5 mg to 50 mg of iodine a day (those with diabetes took 100 mg/day). Patients reported a greater sense of well being, increased energy, lifting of "brain fog," need for less sleep, improved skin complexion, more regular bowel movements, feeling warmer in cold environments, reversal of fibrocystic disease, less need for insulin for diabetics, hypothyroid patients needing less thyroid medication, migraine relief and relief of fibromyalgia symptoms. Although the results are not yet conclusive, they also noted a reduction in the incidence of breast cancer.(86) The authors say that it's hard to overdose on iodine, and ingestion of up to 5 grams a day have shown no ill effects for short periods. But, some people are oversensitive to it, so any supplementation should be done under the supervision of a health care professional.

There are different kinds of iodine. The drug-store tincture of iodine should never be taken internally. The forms that can be taken orally are potassium iodide (KI), super-saturated potassium iodide (SSKI), Lugol's solution (a combination of iodide and iodine, which some doctors think is better than taking iodide alone), Iodoral (Lugol's solution in pill form), and nascent iodine (an atomic from rather than the molecular form the other forms are in – supposedly easier to absorb). Again, only take iodine supplements under the supervision of a health care professional since too much can cause hyperthyroidism and goiter although overdosing is rare. Also, if you have had a history of goiter or other thyroid problems, or are currently taking thyroid medication, only take iodine supplements under a doctor's care.

A simple, but not that precise way to see if you're low on iodine is to do the iodine patch-test. Get a bottle or Tincture of Iodine (the original orange-colored solution, not the clear solution and not *Povidone* Solution) from the drug store.

Warning: Do NOT take this internally. This is NOT the same as SSKI or Lugol's Solution, so do not use it the same way. Tincture of Iodine is for external use only!

Paint a patch of it an inch wide by about 3 inches long on the underside of your forearm or on your abdomen or inner thigh. Do this right before you go to bed. In the morning, look at the patch and notice if there's any color left – it may be grayish, yellow or bright yellow orange (like when you first painted it). If there's no color left at all, then you are definitely iodine deficient. If there's color left, observe it during the day to see if and when it leaves. The quicker it leaves, the more deficient in iodine you are. If all the color isn't gone by bedtime, you're not iodine deficient.

You can also get the iodine-loading test done that is much more accurate. It involves taking a dose of iodine and seeing how much is excreted the next morning. You can order the test kit for this from FFP Labs at (877) 900-5556 or www.helpmythyroid.com (828) 684-3233.

Foods rich in iodine include seafood, vegetables grown in iodine rich soils, seaweeds of all kinds, milk (sometimes), yogurt, eggs, strawberries and raw sunflower seeds. The best source to get iodine is from wild-caught saltwater fish and shellfish. You can figure that 4 - 6 ounces of fish per day will supply you with about half the RDA of 150 mcg. About 2 grams of iodized salt will supply the RDA. Another good source of iodine is seaweeds (kelp, dulse, nori). However, these are also sometimes high in arsenic (which is bad), and have a high salt content. So if you think you might need more iodine, supplementation may be the best way to go. Remember, many researchers consider the iodine RDA too low, so you probably need more in your diet.

Certain foods contain *goitrogenic* compounds – so named because they encourage goiter by blocking the absorption or utilization of iodine. These include cruciferous vegetables (cabbage, broccoli, Brussels sprouts and such), soybean products, peanuts, mustard and millet. So if you're trying to increase your iodine, or you have thyroid problems, cutting back on these foods is advisable. Cooking these foods is believed to eliminate their goitrogenic effects.

Iodine metabolism is dependant on the trace mineral selenium, (discussed in the chapter on the prostate gland in *Everlasting Health*), so adequate supplies of it must be available. Vitamin A, E, and zinc deficiencies can exacerbate the effects of iodine deficiency. So you can see that a nutrient dense diet is necessary to ensure iodine utilization. Some drugs and food coloring agents also have a negative effect iodine metabolism.

Severe iodine deficiency during pregnancy or infancy causes cretinism, a condition characterized by hypothyroidism. This can lead to the failure of the thyroid gland or severe mental retardation, stunted physical growth, deafness, and spasticity. If discovered in its initial stages, cretinism can be corrected with iodine supplementation.

Breast milk contains iodine and lactating women require extra iodide. Dr. Flechas believes that since iodine is so important to the developing fetus and for the first three years of life, the mother should supplement her diet during pregnancy and, if nursing, for the first two years after pregnancy.[87] Goiter or thyroid nodules can be detected with a thyroid ultrasound.

Food for Thought

Iodine consumption in the U.S. has plummeted over the last 30 years. This is chiefly due to two factors:

One: Since 1924, iodine has been added to regular table salt (providing 76 mcg of iodine per gram of salt) to decrease the number of people getting goiter (disease of the thyroid gland). But over the last 25 years, those who use iodized table salt have decreased their consumption of it by 65 percent due to concerns that salt raises blood pressure. In addition, about 45 percent of American households buy salt without iodine added and some health-conscious people now buy sea salt, which, surprisingly contains only trace amounts of iodine. So if you use sea salt, you need to get your iodine somewhere else. Since vegetables grown on land only contain trace amounts of iodine (0.001 mg/g vs. 0.5-8.0 mg/g in marine plants), and there is insufficient iodine in meat and dairy, so supplementation is warranted. The kinds of diets that may cause iodine deficiency are diets without ocean fish or sea vegetables, diets without enough iodized salt, diets high in bakery products that contain bromide (see below), and vegan and vegetarian diets. It's interesting to note that salt restrictive diets are more prevalent in the elderly and that 25 percent of the people over age 60 will become senile as a result of hypothyroidism, which, you know, may be a result of iodine deficiency. So people in the very age group that needs iodine the most may be being told to avoid the condiment that usually supplies it.

Two: In the 1960s and 1970s iodine was added to commercial baking products as a dough conditioned, but in the 1980s it was replaced with bromine due to concerns the high levels of iodine (there was about 150 mcg of iodine in one slice of bread) would cause malfunctioning of the thyroid gland. But there's a problem with that: Bromine (in a class of elements called *halogens*, as are iodine, chlorine, and fluorine), competes with iodine in the body so it interferes with iodine utilization in the thyroid as well as wherever else iodine is used and concentrated (e.g. breast tissue). For this reason, bromine is known as a goitrogen (promotes the formation of goiter). Not good.

Bromine is itself a toxic substance that the body has absolutely no use for and, is a known carcinogen to the breast. And yet they add it to bakery products??? Come on. And men, don't think you're immune from the ravages of iodine deficiency. Dr. Brownstein says that iodine deficiency is a major cause of prostate cancer in American men. The same pattern of cancer of the prostate in Japanese men vs. American men is similar to that of breast cancer in Japanese women vs. American women; and Japanese men who move to the U.S. start getting prostate cancer just like the American men.[88]

Bromine (or in its reduced form of bromide) is pretty nasty stuff. It can cause you to feel dull and apathetic and make it difficult to concentrate, causes depression, headaches, and irritability. It's used to fumigate crops, as an antibacterial agent for pools and hot tubs and used to kill termites and other pests.

Besides being used in the baking industry, it's also used in the production of vegetable oils (brominated vegetable oils), which are oftentimes used in soft drinks and sports drinks. In fact, bromine toxicity has been reported from the ingestion of *Mountain Dew, AMP Energy Drink*, and some *Gatorade* products.(89) Doesn't anyone at the FDA read these reports??? How can something that's used to kill boll weevils and termites be allowed in sports drinks and soda pop? And we wonder why our youth can't get motivated to do anything. One more thing on bromine – it once was used in many medicines, but was removed because of its known toxicity. But it's still in some medicines to treat asthma (inhalers) and bladder dysfunction. Go figure.

Fluoride is another halogen that is very bad for you. (See more in *Everlasting Health*.) It also competes with iodine, so it can cause thyroid problems. It's a major ingredient in antidepressants such as *Paxil*, and it's been documented that women on the SSRI antidepressants that use fluoride have in increased risk of breast cancer.(90)

That's not to mention that fluoride is added to our water supply, toothpaste and mouthwash under the mistaken belief that it strengthens teeth. Instead, it's helping to create an iodine deficiency that's leading to epidemics in breast and prostate cancer.

While we're at it, we might as well look at the last halogen on the list, chlorine. Now *chloride*, is abundant in the body: There's a lot of it naturally in the extra cellular fluid, and it's needed to help break down protein during digestion. But *chlorine* is toxic, and has been linked to birth defects, cancer, reproductive disorders and immune system breakdown.(91) (See *Everlasting Health* for more on this subject.) Since our drinking water is treated with chlorine to disinfect it, we're exposed to it quite often. If that's not enough, you can always get more of this yummy toxic compound by using *Splenda* (sucralose), the sugar-substitute that is nothing but chlorinated table sugar. (The manufacturers of this poison joyously proclaim in their ads – "It's NOT sugar!" No, it's even worse. At least sugar hasn't had an extremely toxic substance added to it!)

Some other good things about iodine: Iodine is a potent anti-oxidant, much along the lines of vitamin C. Iodine induces apoptosis, which is programmed cell death. Why is that good? Because when cells keep growing uncontrollably without dying in their normal lifecycle as they should, cancer results. So iodine is an anti-cancer agent.

Iodine removes toxic chemicals and biological toxins from the body. It rids the body of toxic fluoride and bromide, and even mercury and other heavy metals.(92) Iodine is needed by the main thyroid hormones, T_3 and T_4, and if there isn't enough of it, hypothyroidism will result. Oftentimes, reversing an iodine deficiency can correct a hypothyroid condition. Albert Szent Gyorgi (1983-1986), the physician who discovered vitamin C and winner of the Nobel Prize, has said, "When I was a medical student, iodine in the form of KI was the universal medicine. Nobody knew what it did, but it did something and did something good. We students used to sum up the situation in this little rhyme: If ye don't know where, what, and why . . . Prescribe ye then K and I"

Doctors used to prescribe iodine for many diseases, and in large doses. The 11th edition of the *Encyclopedia Britannica* published in 1911 stated regarding iodine salts (like potassium iodide), ". . . they possess the power of driving out impurities from the blood and tissues. Most notably is this the case with the poisonous products of syphilis. This disease yields in the most rapid and unmistakable fashion to iodides, so much so that the administration of these salts is at present the best means of determining whether, for instance, a cranial tumor be syphilitic or not."(93)

Doctors used to use potassium iodide in doses starting at 1.5 gm to 3 gm and even up to 10 gm a day. Gram amounts of KI are still being used by dermatologists to treat inflammatory dermatoses. They start with an iodine dose of 900 mg/day, followed by weekly increases up to 6 grams a day as tolerated. Side effects of too much iodine generally don't happen, and if they do, are mild: acne, metallic taste in mouth, sneezing, excess saliva and frontal sinus pressure. Always be sure to check with your doctor before making any changes in supplementation or diet.

Remember the ways to tell if you actually need iodine: the simple patch test described above, and a lab test you can get via Jorge D. Flechas, M.D. It costs about $90 and involves a urine sample. To order go to www.helpmythyroid.com or call (828) 684-3233. For more on iodine, I recommend the book by Dr. Brownstein, *Iodine: Why You Need It, Why You Can't Live Without It.*

Maybe we need more iodine than the typical diet supplies. Maybe it can help you avoid breast cancer, prostate cancer (as we'll see in the prostate cancer section), fibrocystic breast disease, or hypothyroidism. Maybe something so simple – supplying the body with the raw materials it needs to function properly – is all we need to do to stay healthy.

Diet

Broccoli, Brussels sprouts, kale and cauliflower contain a compound that can inhibit the growth of cancer cells, including breast cancer. It's been shown that organically grown vegetables contain higher levels of the cancer-fighting class of compounds called flavonoids. This was reported in the *Journal of Agricultural and Food Chemistry*, the *Journal of the American Chemical Society*, the world's largest scientific society.(94,95)

There's evidence that women who consume foods rich in omega-3 fatty acids over many years may be less likely to develop breast cancer, and the risk of dying from breast cancer may be significantly less for those who eat a lot of omega-3s from fish and brown kelp seaweed (common in Japan). The research shows that the balance between omega-3 and omega-6 fatty acids (which should be 2:1) is an important role in the development and growth of breast cancer. Eating fish or taking a good fish oil supplement certainly can't hurt.

As with any cancer and any condition of ill-health, sugar in any shape or form should be avoided. In addition, consumption of a lot of sweet or starch food all at once causes a spike in insulin secretion, which is thought to accelerate the growth of breast cancer cells. Cinnamon has a positive effect on blood sugar levels. So even though there's been no research on cinnamon as far as breast cancer is concerned, it stands to reason that if a spike in insulin accelerates the growth of breast cancer cells, consuming cinnamon might help in this regard. Garlic also has been shown to retard breast cancer growth. A study in France reported in the *European Journal of Epidemiology* showed breast cancer risks for 345 women decreased the more they consumed garlic and onions.(96)

There have been claims that soy offers protection against breast cancer. But the soy plant may be good for fixing nitrogen in soil, but nature didn't intend humans to eat its beans in any shape or form (tofu, hydrolyzed vegetable protein). An article in the *Journal of Nutrition*, reported there were no significant differences in breast tissue density (an increase in breast tissue density is associated with increased risk for breast cancer) between women who consumed soy regularly over a two year period and those who didn't. In fact, women who consumed more soy during their lives had a higher percentage densities than women whose diet included little soy.(97)

Researchers have reported that women who ate flame-broiled meat more than twice a month had an increased risk of developing breast cancer. Not just that, but women who consumed the most well-done meat compared to those who ate less-cooked meat were twice as likely to develop breast cancer.(98) The problem comes from cooking meat at high temperatures (by any method), and by charring the meat during grilling. Charred meat contains heterocyclic amines, which are believed to promote many types of cancer, not just breast cancer.

A study at the Harvard Medical School said that giving girls under five years old one portion of chips (fried) increases their risk of developing breast cancer later in life by 27 percent. Deep frying is the culprit here, so I'm sure that French fries (a favorite food of kids), would probably do the same thing.(99)

It's also thought that breast tissue is especially vulnerable to damage from the carcinogens in tobacco smoke during puberty when breast cells are actively dividing. Second hand smoke exposure during this time may increase the risk of breast cancer later.

Exercise

Exercise is important to avoid breast cancer, if you have breast cancer, and recovering from breast cancer. One study of 65,000 women showed that high levels of physical activity from ages 12 to 22 had a 23 percent lower risk of getting breast cancer risk before menopause (one-quarter of all breast cancers are diagnosed in women before menopause). The lead investigator Graham Colditz, M.D., Dr. P.H said, "We don't have a lot of prevention strategies for premenopausal breast cancer, but our findings clearly show that physical activity during adolescence and young adulthood can pay off in the long run by reducing a woman's risk of early breast cancer."(100)

Another study showed that women who have had breast cancer and walk or did the equivalent of walking at a pace of 2-3 mph improve their survival rate (compared to inactive women) depending on how long they exercised: one to three hours/week resulted in a 20 percent lower death rate; three to five hours/week decreased the risk of death by 50 percent, and five to eight hours/week resulted in a decrease in death rate of 44 percent. After 10 years, of the women who exercised about half an hour per day (three to five hours per week), 92 percent were still alive. Of those who got less than an hour a week, only 86 percent were still alive.(101,102)

Two of the best exercises you can do to help avoid breast cancer is swimming (try to do it in water that is not chlorinated) and arm circles (hold your arms out like you're flying and circle them around). This is because these exercises move the areas right next to your arm pits where major lymph glands are. As you move these areas, the lymph circulates better and any toxins in these areas are removed. Breast cancer is much more serious when it spreads into the lymph glands, so doing these exercises greatly improves your chances of avoiding the cancer or reversing it, and it may help counteract the effects of wearing a bra.

Breast Implants and Breast Cancer

Currently, about 300,000 women a year (about two million since it started in 1962), have had breast augmentation surgery. Eighty percent of these surgeries are for purely cosmetic reasons, while 20 percent are for breast reconstruction after breast cancer. The first implants used in 1962 when this surgery began, were filled with silicone. So many problems occurred with them that the leading manufacturer at the time, Dow Corning Corp. faced 19,000 lawsuits related to their silicone implants, resulting in its filing for Chapter 11 bankruptcy in 1995.

Subsequently, silicone implants were banned by the FDA, being replaced with saline ones. But in 2006, the FDA reversed its stance and has approved them for use in women over the age of 22. Dr. Sidney Wolfe, who works for Public Citizen, a national non-profit public interest organization, said, "In terms of adverse safety and health information known at the time of approval–such as high rates of rupture, the need for repeat surgery and clear evidence of lymph node infiltration and damage by leaked silicone–silicone gel breast implants are the most defective medical device ever approved by the FDA. The approval makes a mockery of the legal standard that requires 'reasonable assurance of safety'" (103)

But do breast implants cause breast cancer? They do interfere with mammograms, preventing about 10 percent of the tissue to be adequately scanned. (Of course, you should never get a mammogram, but use thermography or sonography instead.) The pressure exerted on the implant during the test may in fact rupture the implant.

It appears that there's no real difference in breast cancer incidences or mortality between women who have breast implants and those who don't.(104,105) But this research also showed that women who have had the surgery (strictly for cosmetic reasons), had two to three times higher rates for brain and respiratory cancers.(106) Another study of 23,500 women found that women with breast implants had a suicide rate 73 percent higher than women in the general population.(107) The researchers think that the high suicide rate is due to the type of women who gets the surgery, not to the implants: the psychological profile of women who receive breast implants is characterized by lack of self-confidence, low self-esteem and more frequent mental illnesses such as depression.

Special Section:
The common Food Everyone Eats that Makes Cancer Cells Spread

One of the worst things you can put in your mouth as far as cancer is concerned, is sugar. It's a major food for cancer cells. In fact, cancer cells thrive on it. Is this a new discovery? No. In 1931 Dr. Otto Warburg was awarded the Nobel Prize for discovering that cancer cells thrive on sugar. This is because cancer cells metabolize through fermentation, and fermentation requires sugar. Fermentation is an anaerobic process (no oxygen involved), unlike normal respiration that requires oxygen. So it's not surprising that cancer cells hate oxygen. In fact, a popular alternative cancer therapy is oxygen therapy where the body is flooded with oxygen. Dr. Warburg found that he could create cancer by lowering the oxygen content in a cell to 35 percent and, he could reverse cancer by increasing the oxygen content. (See the chapter on asthma in *Everlasting Health* for a breathing method that will get more oxygen to your cells – and it's NOT deep breathing!) So healthy cells get their energy from oxygen, cancer cells get theirs from fermentation which requires sugar.[108] Eating sugar just encourages cancer to form, and if you have it already, to flourish.

Sugar causing cancer is not just theory. A study reported in the *Journal of the National Cancer Institute* shows that women who consumed a high glycemic load diet (a diet high in carbohydrates, sucrose, and fructose – i.e. sugars) were nearly three times more likely to develop colon cancer.[109]

In a study of 80,000 men and women between 1997 and 2005, those who drank soft drinks at least twice a day had a 90 percent higher risk of developing pancreatic cancer than those who didn't drink them at all. People who added sugar to food or drinks (like coffee) at least five times a day had a 70 percent higher risk of this cancer.[110] So cut down and eliminate sugar, and you'll greatly cut down on your chances of getting cancer.

Another thing that cancer loves you to do is to eat cooked foods. This is again related to oxygen. Cooking destroys not only a lot of vitamins, but it also destroys enzymes. Enzymes are needed by the body for a multitude of reasons, one of which relates to how red blood cells clump together. If the enzymes aren't there, the blood cells will clump more, and won't be able to fit through tiny microcapillaries. This causes many anaerobic (low or no oxygen) areas in the body, thus encouraging cancer. To avoid or reverse cancer, it's best to stop eating sugar (all starch based carbohydrates like pasta, breads, etc., are essentially made of two sugar molecules bound together), and cooked foods. See *Everlasting Health* for more on sugar.

References

1. www.breastcancer.org.
2. www.cancer.org.
3. Sherman, Janette D, *Life's Delicate Balance; The Causes and Prevention of Breast Cancer*, New York and London: Taylor and Francis, 2000.
4. American Cancer Society.
5. Hanse NM, et al. "Manipulation fo the Primary Breast Tumor and the Incidence of Sentinel Node Metastases from Invasive Breast Cancer." Arch Surg. 2004;139:634-640.
6. www.cancer.org.
7. Douglass, WC, Real Health Breakthroughs, Vol 5 No. 10, March 2006.
8. Cancer statistics, 2004. *Cancer. Clin.* 2004;54:8-29.
9. www.alternativemedicine.com.
10. Miller AB, Baines CJ, Wall C, "Canadian National Breast Screening Study-2: 13-year Results of a Randomized Trial in Women Aged 50-59 Years." *J Natl Cancer Inst*, 2000 Sep 20;92(18):1490-9.
11. Miller AB, Baines CJ, Wall C, "Mammograms in Women Age 40 to 49: Results of the Canadian Breast Cancer Screening Study." *Annals of Internal Medicine*. 3 Sept 2002 Vol 137, Issue 5, Part 1, Page 1-28.
12. Miller, AB et al. "Canadian National Breast Screening Study-2: 13-Year Results of a Randomized Trial in Women Aged 50-59 Year." *Journal of the National Cancer Institute*. September 20, 2000; 92:1490-1499.
13. www.mercola.com.
14. Northstar Nutritionals newsletter, 12/11/2008.

15. Zahl et al. "The Natural History of Invasive Breast Cancers Detected by Screening Mammography." Arch Intern Med. 2008;168(21):2302-2303
16. *The Lancet*, July 11, 1992.
17. www.nci.gov.
18. www.nih.gov.
19. NewsTarget.com, August 15, 2005.
20. *The Daily Dose*, Douglass, WC, Feb 17, 2004.
21. Ibid.
22. Personal Communication, Tracy Cousins, M.D., Wausau, WI
23. *The Lancet*, July 11, 1992, p. 122
24. Douglass, Op cit.
25. Gofman, JohnW. Preventing Breast Cancer, Committee for Nuclear Responsibility; 2nd edition, Feb. 1996.
26. Cochrane Database Syst Rev. 2001:(4):CD001877, Cochrane Database Syst Rev. 2006:(4):CD001877.
27. Wright CJ, Mueller CB, "Screening Mammography and Public Health Policy." *The Lancet*, July 1995.
28. Caplan A. "Breast Cancer Tests - Not Worth the Price" MSNBC Oct. 8, 2008.
29. Parikh YR et al. "Efficacy of Computerized Infrared Imaging Analysis to Evaluate Mammographically Suspicious Lesions." *American J Roentgenolgy*. 180 (2003):263-269.
30. Gamagami P. "Indirect Signs of Breast Cancer: Angiogenesis Study." *Atlas of Mammography*, Cambridge, MA, Blackwell Science pp 231-26, 1996.
31. Okihara K et al. "Transrectal Power Doppler Imaging in the Detection of Prostate Cancer." British Journal of Urology. June 2000
32. www.cancerscan.com and *AmericanJournalofRadiolog*. January, 2000
33. "What Causes Breast Cancer?" *Rachel's Environment & Health News*, #723 - April 26, 2001.
34. Westin, Jerome B., and Elihu Richter. "The Israeli Breast-Cancer Anomaly." In *Trends in Cancer Mortality in Industrial Countries*, edited by Devra L. Davis and David Hoel. New York: Academy of Sciences, 1990, pp 259-268.
35. Montague, Peter. "Breast Cancer Epidemic Continues; Prevention Philosophy is Ignored," *Rachel's Environmental & Health Weekly*. Environmental Research Foundation. December 25, 1991.
36. Montague, Peter. "Human Breast Milk is Contaminated," *Rachel's Environmental & Health Weekly*. Environmental Research Foundation. August 8, 1990.
37. Foster, Warren, et. al. "In Utero Exposure of the Human Fetus to Xenobiotic Endocrine Disrupting Chemicals." Presented at the Endocrine Society's 81st Annual Meeting in San Diego, CA, June 14, 1999.
38. Davis, Devra L., et al. "Medical Hypothesis: Xenoestrogens as Preventable Causes of Breast Cancer." *Environmental Health Perspectives* 101 (October 1993):372-377.
39. Montague, Peter. "Chemicals and Health – Part 1." Rachel's Environmental & Health Weekly. Environmental Research Foundation. December 23, 1993.
40. National Institutes of Health - National Heart, Lung and Blood Institute Press Release, "NHLB Stops Trial of Estrogen Plus Progestin Due to Increased Breast Cancer Risk, Lack of Overall Benefit." July 9, 2002.
41. www.nlm.nih.gov/medlineplus/print/ency/article/007111.htm.
42. www.equineadvocates.com.
43. www.mercola.com.
44. Writing Group for the Women's Health Initiative Investigators. "Risk and Benefits of Estrogen Plus Progestin in Healthy Postmenopausal Women: Principal Results from the Women's Health Initiative Randomized Controlled Trial. *JAMA*. 2002; 288:321-333.
45. "Breast Cancer Drop Tied to Less Hormone Therapy." MSNBC News Services, Dec 14, 2006.
46. Sherman Janett D. *Life's Delicate Balance; The Causes and Prevention of Breast Cancer*. New York and London: Taylor and Francis, 2000
47. Cone, M., "Banned Elsewhere, Compounds Still Used in U.S." *LA Times*, October 8, 2006
48. Sherman JD. Op cit.
49. Eliassen AH, et al. "Adult Weight Change and Risk of Post-menopausal Breast Cancer." *JAMA*. 2006;296:193-201.
50. Darbre, PD. "Underarm Cosmetics and Breast Cancer." *Journal of Applied Toxicology*, 2003. Mar-Apr;23(2):89-05.
51. McGrath, K. "An Earlier Age of Breast Cancer Diagnosis Related to More Frequent Use of Antiperspirants/deodorants and Underarm Shaving." *European Journal of Cancer Prevention*, Vol. 12, p. 479.
52. www. breastcancerfund.com.
53. Velicer CM, et al. "Antibiotic use in Relation to the Risk of Breast Cancer." *JAMA*, Feb. 18, 2004;291(7):827-35.
54. Marshall, SF, et al. "Nonsteroidal Anti-Inflammatory Drug Use and Breast Cancer Risk by Stage and Hormone Receptor Status." *Journal of the National Cancer Institute*. June 1, 2005, Vol. 97, No.11:805-812.
55. Cotterchio, M. et al. "Antidepressant Medication Use and Breast Cancer Risk." *American Journal of Epidemiology*, May 2000 151:951-957.
56. 35th Annual Meeting of the Society for Epidemiologic Research, Seattle, June 2000.
57. *BBC News*, Jan. 7, 2004.
58. www.breakthechain.org.
59. Ibid.
60. Bromfield, L. *Pleasant Valley*. Wooster Book Company, 1997.
61. Grant WB. "An Estimate of Premature Cancer Mortality in the U.S. due to Inadequate Doses of Solar Ultraviolet-B Radiation." Cancer. 2002;94:1867-1875.
62. Garland, et al. *Prev Med*. 1990;19:614-622.
63. Lamson, C. "Suggestions that Vitamin D May Protect against Breast Cancer (AACR Annual Meeting). " *Oncology Times*. Vol 28(12)25 June 2006 p 50-51.
64. American Association of Cancer Research Annual Meeting, Washington, DC, April 1-6, 2006.
65. Lowe LC, et al. "Plasma 25-hydroxy Vitamin D Concentrations, Vit D Receptof Genotype and Breast Cancer Risk in a UK Caucasian Population." *Eur J Cancer*. 2005;41:1164-1169
66. Bertone-Johnson ER, et al. "Plasma 25-Hydroxyvitamin D and 1,25-Dihydroxyvitamin D and Risk of Breast Cancer" Cancer Epidemiol Biomarkers. Prev. 2005;14:1991-1997.
67. Laino, Charlene. Vitamin D may protect against cancer. WebM.D. April 4, 2006.
68. Sircus, M. *Transdermal Magnesium Therapy*. 2007. Phaelos Books, Chandler AZ.
69. Werbach, M. M.D., *J Alt & Comp Med*. Feb. 1994;12(2)
70. Sircus, M., Op cit.
71. Eskin, BA. "Iodine and Mammary Cancer." Tanscript, NY Acadamy of Sciences. 1970
72. Drouse, T. Age-related changes in iodine-blocked. Proc. Amer. Ass. Cancer Research. 18. 1977
73. Brownstein, D. *Iodine, Why you need it why you can't live without it*. Medical Alternatives Press, W. Bloomfield, MI. 2008.
74. Eskin, BA. "Mammary gland dysplasia in iodine deficiency." *JAMA*. May 22, 1967.
75. Brownstein, D., Op Cit.
76. Finley, JW et al. "Breast Cancer and Thyroid Disease." *Quart. Rev. Surg. Obstet. and Gyn*. 1960 17:139
77. Miller, Jr., DW. "Extrathyroidal Benefits of Iodine," *Journal of American Physicians and Surgeons*. Vol. 11, No. 4, Winter 2006.
78. Cann SA, van Netten JP, van Netten C. "Hypothesis: Iodine, Selenium and the Development of Breast Cancer." *Cancer Causes Control*. 2000;11:121-127.
79. Eskin BA, et al. "Identification of Breast Cancer by Differences in Urinary Iodine." *Proc Am Assoc Cancer Res*. 2005;46:504.
80. Bogardus, AG. *Surgery*. 1960, 49, 461. and Finley, J. rev. *Obstet. Gynec*. 1960, 49, 17.
81. Beaston, G. "Adjuvant Use of Thyroid Extract in Breast Cancer." *Lancet*. 104:no.2,pg.162,1896.
82. Vishniakova YY, Murav'eva NI. "On the Treatment of Dyshormonal Hyperplasia of Mammary Glands." *Vestn Akad Nauk* (USSR) Russian, 1966;21(9);19-22.
83. Ghent WR, Eskin BA, Low DA, Hill LP. "Iodine Replacement in Fibrocystic Disease of the Breast." *Can. J. Surg*. 1993;36-453-460.
84. Kessler JH. "The Effect of Supraphysiologic Levels of Iodine on Patients with Cyclic Mastalgia." *Breast J*. 2004;10:328-336.
85. Brownstein, D., Op cit.
86. Miller, Jr. Op cit.
87. www.helpmythyroid.com .
88. Ibid.
89. Horowitz, B. "Bromism from Excessive Cola Consumption." *Clinical Toxicology*, 35(3)(315-320. 1997.
90. 35th Annual Meeting of the Society for Epidemiologic Research, Seattle, WA June, 2000.
91. Cantor KP, Hildesheim ME, Lynch CF, et al. "Drinking Water Source and Chlorination Byproducts: Risk of Bladder Cancer." *Epidemiology*. 1998:9(part 1):21-28. and; Hildesheim ME, Cantor KP, Lynch CF, et al. "Drinking Water Source and Chlorination Byproducts: Risk of Colon and Rectal Cancers." Epidemiology 1998;9(part 2):29-35. *Epidemiology*. May 1999. 10:233-237.
92. Brownstein, op cit.
93. Miller, DW Jr., *Iodine for Health*. Lewrockwell.com
94. Journal of Biological Chemistry. June 6, 2003.
95. "Organically Grown Foods Higher in Cancer-fighting Chemicals than Conventionally Grown Foods." *ScienceDaily*, Mar. 4, 2003. and Asami DK, et al. "Comparison of the Total Phenolic and Ascorbic Acid Content of Freeze-dried and Air-dried Marionberry, Strawberry, and Corn Grown using Conventional Organic, and Sustainable Agricultural Practices." *Journal of Agricultural and Food Chemistry*. Feb. 26 2003 51(5);1237-41.
96. Challier B, Perarnau JM, Viel JF. "Garlic, Onion and Cereal Fibre as Protective Factors for Breast Cancer: A French case-control study. *European Journal of Epidemiology* 1998; 14(8):737-747.
97. Maskarinec G, et al. "A 2-year Soy Intervention in Premenopausal Women Does Not Change Mammographic Densities. *Journal of Nutrition*, Nov. 2004; 134:3089-3094.
98. Annual Meeting of the American Association for Cancer Research. April 3, 2000
99. Macrae, Fiona, "Frying Can Increase Cancer Risk." Mail Online, www.dailymail.co.uk. April 10, 2006.
100. Arbanas, C. "Girls, Young Women Can Cut Risk of Early Breast Cancer Through Regular Exercise," Washington University School of Medicine, Press Release, May 13, 2008
101. Holmes, M.D., et al., "Physical Activity and Survival after Breast Cancer Diagnosis." *JAMA*. May 25, 2005:293:2479-2486.
102. www.cancer.org.
103. *Newsinferno.com*. "FDA Lifts 14-Year Ban on Silicone Breast Implants," November 20, 2006.
104. Brinton LA, et al. "Breast Cancer Following Augmentation Mammoplasty,(U.S.)" *Cancer Causes & Control* 2000;11(9):819-827.
105. Brinton LA et al. "Cancer Risk at Sites other than Breast Following Augmentation Mammoplasty." *Annals of Epidemiology*. May 2001;11(4):248-256.
106. Brinton, LA et al. "Mortality among Augmentation Mammoplasty Patients." *Epidemiology*. May 2001;12(3):321-326.
107. Villeneuve, PJ, et al. "Mortality among Canadian Women with Cosmetic Breast Implants." *American Journal of Epidemiology*. 2006. 164(4):334-341, August 15, 2006.
108. www.hopeforcancer.com
109. Higginbotham, S. et al. "Dietary Glycemic Load and Risk of Colorectal Cancer in the Women's Health Study." *Journal of the National Cancer Institute*, February 4, 2004;96(3):229-233.
110. Larsson, SC, Bergkvist, L., Wolk, A. "Consumption of Sugar and Sugar-sweetened Foods and the Risk of Pancreatic Cancer in a Prospective Study." *American Journal of Clinical Nutrition*, November 2006; 84(5): 1171-1176

Prostate Cancer, BPH, & Better Sex for Men

11 Natural & Money-saving Ways to Improve Prostate Health

Introduction

The prostate gland is a small gland that's part of the male reproductive system. It secretes much of the liquid portion of semen, the milky fluid that transports sperm through the penis during ejaculation. It's located just below the bladder in front of the rectum, and encircles a section of the urethra (the tube that carries urine from the bladder out the penis). During ejaculation, semen is secreted by the prostate through small pores in the walls of the urethra.

Interestingly, the prostate gland is in a continual state of growth throughout a man's life. So it's not surprising that the older the man, the more the prostate will be a problem. In young men, the prostate gland is usually healthy and not large enough to cause problems. The three most common prostate problems are inflammation (prostatitis), prostatic enlargement (benign prostatic hyperplasia or BPH), and prostate cancer.

Inflammation of the prostate causes it to enlarge. Not surprisingly, prostatitis can cause difficult or painful urination that feels like burning, and a strong and frequent urge to urinate, which results in only small amounts of urine sometimes accompanied by pain in the lower back or abdomen.

Benign Prostatic Hyperplasia (BPH)

BPH is an enlarged prostate due to excessive growth of tissue. This tissue is noncancerous, or benign, and why it occurs is still not known. By age 60, more than half of all American men have at least microscopic signs of BPH. By age 70, more than 40 percent will have enlargement that can be felt on physical examination.[1]

A man with BPH finds it hard to initiate the flow of urine, and it may be just a dribble. He may need to urinate frequently or have a sudden, powerful urge to urinate. He likely has to get up several times a night to urinate, or have the feeling that the bladder is never completely empty. Straining to empty the bladder is not advisable, since it can harm the muscular walls of the bladder and damage the kidneys. BPH can eventually weaken the bladder, and once the bladder is damaged, it's virtually impossible to repair. A weak bladder can lead to other complications such as bladder stones and bleeding. In severe cases, the man may need to be catheterized; a procedure in which a tube called a catheter is inserted through the penis into the bladder to allow urine to escape.

The prostate in a healthy young male is about the size of a walnut. By the time a man is 40 years old, the prostate may already have grown to the size of an apricot. By age 60, it could be as big as a lemon. One doctor said, "You know the old saying about death and taxes – two things in this life we can be sure of. But for American men age 50 and over, I must, unfortunately add another certainty: prostate problems."[2]

BPH is detected by a physical exam called a "digital rectal examination" where the doctor inserts his finger up the rectum to feel the elasticity and size of the prostate. The source of many locker-room jokes, it's not a fun experience. Urinalysis is done to check for bleeding or infection, and a blood test called a prostate-specific antigen (PSA) test may be run to see if cancer of the prostate is present. Oftentimes, X-rays, and ultrasound may be used, although according to federal guidelines, these add nothing to the decision as to what form of treatment should be used. These tests, although unnecessary, are routinely used by two-thirds of urologists, which add up to tens of millions of dollars every year.[3]

About half of the men with BPH develop symptoms serious enough to warrant treatment. But consider that BPH is not an indication of or precursor to prostate cancer, and it doesn't increase your chances of prostate cancer either. We'll examine ways to improve prostate health towards the end of this handbook. But for now, some remedial actions to take include limiting fluid intake in the evening, especially beverages that contain alcohol or caffeine, taking time to empty the bladder completely when urinating, and not allowing long intervals to pass without urinating. Another helpful thing to know is that over-the-counter cold and flu medicines can cause increased urinary retention, hindering the ability to urinate, so it's best to avoid them.[4]

Medical treatments for serious cases of BPH include drugs and surgery. Drug therapy for BPH started in the early 1990s. There are two classes of drugs that can increase urine flow, but in different ways.

Alpha adrenergic blockers (or alpha-1 blockers), originally used for the treatment of high blood pressure, relax smooth muscles in the muscular portion of the prostate and the area where the urethra comes out of the bladder. Generic drug names are phenoxybenzamine, prazosin, tamsulosin hydrochloride (*Flomax*), and terazosin. Side effects include dizziness, fatigue, and headaches. One of these drugs, trade name *Hytrin* (terazosin), is being prescribed, but there's no knowledge of its long-term effects. But since alpha adrenergic blockers have been used for some time now for the treatment of high blood pressure, we do know one of their ugly side effects – impotence. If your blood pressure is normal and you take a drug that lowers blood pressure, then the drug could cause your blood pressure to drop to a dangerously low level. Other side effects of *Hytrin* are weakness, fatigue, headaches, edema, palpitations, nasal congestion, sleepiness, decreased libido, and blurred vision.

Another class of medicine used for BPH is enzyme inhibitors and include dutasteride (*Avodart*) and finasteride (*Proscar*). They block the enzyme called 5-alpha-reductase, which is necessary to change testosterone (the male sex hormone) into another hormone called dihydrotestosterone, or DHT. It's believed that DHT causes the prostate to enlarge. Merck & Company, its manufacturer, admits that it takes a full 6 months of continual use for this drug to work, and that although it may shrink the prostate, symptoms of BPH may not go away. In addition, once the patient stops using it, its effects wear off, and men who start may have to take this medicine for the rest of their lives.(5) This drug has also been used to stimulate hair growth in men, but at smaller doses.

Typical side effects of *Proscar* and *Avodart* include back pain, decreased libido, decreased volume of semen, diarrhea, rash, itching, hives, dizziness, headache, and impotence. Women are warned to not even handle the pills, since that can cause birth defects in a male fetus (it causes changes in the genitals of the fetus). Another interesting side effect is these drugs may cause a man's breasts to enlarge. A statement on the *Proscar* website says, ". . .some men may have breast enlargement and/or tenderness. You should promptly report to your doctor any changes in your breasts such as lumps, pain, or nipple discharge." (That sounds worse than having to pee every two hours!)

Food for Thought

William Campbell Douglass, M.D. says the following about *Proscar* and the prostate in his report *Prostate Problems: Safe, Simple, Effective Relief. . .*

"But in fact, studies reported in the *New England Journal of Medicine* indicate that *Proscar doesn't work at all.* There is also a possibility that the drug is carcinogenic. Wouldn't that be something? A "cure" approved by the FDA that gives you cancer.

But here's the really sleazy part of this story: Saw palmetto berries, in the form of an extract called LSE seronoa, are just as effective as *Proscar* in inhibiting the conversion of testosterone to DHT, maybe more so. The herb is nontoxic and costs a third as much as *Merck*'s drug. But the Food and Drug Administration rejected an application to have the extract approved as an over-the-counter treatment for BPH. Although the saw palmetto extract has been used for BPH since 1905, and is listed in all the pharmacopeias, the *Physician's Desk Reference* (until 1948, when it was quietly removed), and all the pharmacy texts, the FDA declared the herb to be an "unapproved new drug!". . .

Get some saw palmetto berries and make a tea out of them (weak at first to test your sensitivity, then gradually increase the strength) or make an "infusion"(prolonged soaking in water) and keep it refrigerated. [Be sure you get organically grown berries.] Drink the tea or the infusion, one cupful, three times a day. There is scientific evidence for this treatment. Saw palmetto berries inhibit the enzyme 5-alpha-reductase, and a low activity of this enzyme is associated with a reduced risk of prostate cancer. This berry is also effective in the treatment of benign prostatic hypertrophy, which is not always so benign in its effects."

Dr. Campbell also recommends to empty the bladder as fully as possible when urinating (do not strain, though), avoid long intervals between urination, and to use parsley as a "prostate herbal" and to make a tea of it - "the stronger the better" and add lemon for taste. (Even better, just make some fresh parsley juice using a good juicer.) (6)

According to one herbal website, there have been over a dozen clinical studies involving almost 3,000 men showed that saw palmetto can markedly alleviate BPH symptoms without decreasing the man's libido like prostate drugs do.(7) Saw palmetto is effective in 90 percent of patients suffering from BPH within the first year of treatment compared to less than 50 percent for patients taking finasteride (*Proscar*). And since saw palmetto prevents testosterone from converting to DHP, it has been (anecdotally) reported to stop hair loss and trigger hair growth. There are no known side effects to saw palmetto (it's even OK for women to handle the berries).

The berries were used as food by the Seminole Indians in Florida, and have also been used to ease upset stomachs and insomnia. In the early part of the 20th century, it was commonly recommended as a treatment for BPH and chronic urinary tract infections. It's still being used for prostate problems in Europe, even though here in the U.S., most doctors will probably tell you it's ineffective and recommend the emasculating, poisonous, possibly carcinogenic, drugs.

Prostate Cancer

In the mid-80s, the number of men diagnosed with prostate cancer was about 90,000 per year. By 1997, that figure had risen to an estimated 209,000. In 2006, the number of men being diagnosed with it is around 220,000 per year with 30,000 of them dying from the disease.

The explosion of prostate cancer from the mid-80s to mid-90s is attributed in part to better detection methods. In addition to the digital rectal exam, doctors began using a blood test called the prostate-specific antigen (PSA), which detects a protein produced by prostate cells and is normally present in small quantities in the blood. Often it is elevated when cancer is present, but can also be elevated in some benign disorders of the prostate. – so it's not a foolproof test.(8) It's interesting to note that the researcher who developed the PSA test, is so unhappy with the inaccuracy of his test, that he wishes he had never developed it. He has made this statement due to the fact that a large percentage of men undergo surgery based on their PSA number, only to find out that in fact they do not have prostate cancer. However, a true increase could very well be the case, considering that other degenerative diseases are also on the rise and that one theory of why men get prostate cancer in the first place is because of toxins in our environment – specifically, chemicals and estrogenic pollutants (xenoestrogens). Prostate cancer is the second most prevalent cancer in men (skin cancer is first), and it's estimated that one American male in 10 will get it.(9)

The average age of diagnosis of prostate cancer is age 72. More than 75 percent of prostate cancer cases are in men age 65 or older with only 7 percent occurring in men younger than age 60. African-American men have the world's highest incidence of prostate cancer – a full 33 percent greater than a white American man. Smoking is another risk factor as is eating processed foods. But the actual cause of prostate cancer is presently not known.

Although many men may end up getting prostate cancer, for many of them, it will surface when they are in their 70s and 80s and the cancer is usually slow growing. The Federal Consumer Information Center says a man with the low-grade localized disease "is much more likely to die of other causes than of prostate cancer."(10) In fact, seven out of 10 men diagnosed with prostate cancer (in Canada) die from other causes.(11)

PSA, when elevated above 4ng/mL (nanograms per milliliter), can indicate prostate cancer. This screening test is recommended by the American Cancer Society and the American Urological Association to be performed yearly on men age 50 and over. But other research indicates that anyone with lower PSA levels (below 1.9 ng/ml) the recommendation is to be tested every two years.(12)

As mentioned above, the PSA test is unreliable. There are often false positives and false negatives, so one cannot be sure either way. If a doctor sees a positive high level, he/she may be inclined to treat it with drugs or want to perform surgery, when these may not really be needed. Plus, the doctor may want to poke around to get a biopsy, and this in itself may actually spread the cancer (disturbed cancer cells reproduce faster). Dr. Campbell says, "under no circumstances should you permit your doctor to perform a needle biopsy on the tumor. Such a biopsy can only help to spread the cancer throughout your system. A needle, no matter how small, is basically a knife, and when the needle passes into the gland, it is cutting tissue, which, if cancer is present, can spread the tumor. A cancer that is localized in the prostate is a problem, but it can be controlled. Once the cancer branches out, your chances of survival drop to below 20 percent."(13)

There's a new way to test for prostate cancer that you won't hear about in the mainstream – Power Doppler Sonography (PDS). It's very advanced ultrasound that can produce a detailed image of the body's internal structures and has a much higher resolution and the ability to highlight areas of blood flow in dense or soft tissue, allowing tumors or inflammation to be viewed and measured clearly. In addition, the 3D version of PDS can detest the spread of cancer through the margins of the prostate (or breast in breast cancer). One study reported in the *British Journal of Urology* showed that this kind of screening only misses 1 percent of prostate cancers.(14) Prostate sonograms are safe, painless, and inexpensive. Unlike other screening methods, they can be repeated as often as necessary to closely monitor areas of concern and assess treatment efficacy. For these reasons, sonograms have been found to be a more effective alternative to biopsies in detecting prostate tumors, and better than MRI and PET/CT Scans as a means for tracking these tumors. PDS can also be used to monitor inflammation and tumors in the breast and other parts of the human body (see breast cancer chapter). To learn where you can get a sonogram, check out www.cancerscan.com and www.phoenixsonograms.com.

Food for Thought

The cancerscan.com website is that of Robert L. Bard, M.D., who is one of the best known and highly regarded leaders in the field of sonography. He has experience using sonography in just about every area of the body, and tells me that he can now detect skin cancer (melanoma) and other cancers accurately and early. He is also working to find alternative treatments to treating cancer. Sonography detects 40 percent more invasive cancers than mammograms. When combined with Doppler imaging, it is also excellent at finding the most aggressive tumors that grow so quickly they need a larger blood supply (these are called *interval* cancers).(15) Sonography will become the method of choice in the not-to-distant future for detecting both prostate and breast cancer for several reasons: It is very accurate, it's easy to do and doesn't take long, it's non-invasive, inexpensive and does absolutely no harm to the patient in any way. However, the traditional medical community will be reluctant to switch to it because they make so much money using the other, more profitable diagnostic methods. But eventually, people will wake up and start demanding it.

There are four stages to prostate cancer: A through D. (This is also called the Gleason Curve.)

Stage A: This stage is difficult to diagnose since the number of cancer cells are so few, even with the PSA test. There are no symptoms with this stage, and it's really not worth worrying about. Intervention might do more harm than good.

Stage B: This is when a tumor is present, but it's still confined to the prostate. The symptoms for this stage cancer are the same as BPH, or no symptoms at all.

Stage C: The tumor is no longer confined to the prostate gland, and it likely has spread to the testicles. Symptoms may increase plus pain in the prostate.

Stage D: Here the cancer has metastasized (spread throughout the body). There's pain in the pelvis, lower back and upper thighs.

If a cancer is detected, a prostate acid phosphatase test (PAP), also sometimes called the prostate specific acid phosphatase test (PSAP), may be done to see if the cancer has spread. But unfortunately, this test isn't fool-proof either: 25 percent of patients with stage D prostate cancer have a normal PAP level.(16) If you have Stage C, you need to take action, but not necessarily drugs or surgery.

Food for Thought

Dr. Campbell recommends getting a second and even third opinion on the kind of treatment your doctor recommends if you have prostate cancer, and to get these opinions from doctors in different towns. He says doctors don't want to offend a colleague they know with a different diagnosis. Good advice for any medical situation (and many legal situations too!). He also says not to let a doctor pressure you into quick surgery. Since the vast majority of prostate cancers are slow moving, you should have plenty of time to make a decision or pursue other treatment options. Another doctor who has done extensive investigation into prostate cancer is Isreal Barkin, M.D., F.A.C.S. His website is www.pcref.org.

Prostate Cancer, BPH & Better Sex for Men

Although a standard way to treat prostate cancer in its early stages is with surgery, there's no hard evidence that it's any more effective than waiting and seeing if the condition gets worse (which may include drug therapy). In fact, doing nothing at all seems to be just as effective as surgery or radiation treatments as far as survival rates go, an opinion echoed in the *Journal of the American Medical Association.*(17) That's because prostate cancer is not only slow growing, but usually stays within the confines of the gland itself for many years. Surgery, especially in an old man who probably has other health issues, could be harmful and even fatal due to blood clots or the cancer spreading triggered by the surgery itself.

Prostate surgery can often lead to unwanted problems. Dr. James Talcott found that of 282 patients who had prostate surgery, within a year of their operation, 41 percent of them had to wear diapers because of chronic leaking from their bladder. Other research showed that 60 percent of the men who had prostate surgery were impotent 18 months after the surgery, and 8 percent had complete urinary incontinence. Dr. Talcott says, "Patients need to know what they are in for. We need to prepare them for the bad things that may befall them." Probably, few doctors actually do.(18,19)

This is not to say that surgery is never needed. If the cancer is at Stage C, it may be. Removal of the prostate could save your life (although it will destroy your sex life) and extend it many years. But check out alternative methods first. If you follow the recommendations in this booklet, hopefully, you will never get prostate cancer.

Another form of mainstream treatment is radiation. The main problem radiation is that it kills good cells along with the cancer cells. Nausea, diarrhea, and rectal bleeding may result also. It's another treatment better off avoided.

It's been shown that testosterone, the male sex hormone, encourages the growth of prostate cancer. So testosterone deprivation, or ablation, is used to treat prostate cancer. To do this, the testicles are removed, since testosterone is made in them. Besides the obvious inconveniences of being castrated, this treatment has been shown to negatively affect memory. Interestingly, theories are that lack of testosterone affects the hippocampus – the part of the brain implicated in Alzheimer's disease.(21) On the other hand, some experts note that younger men, who generally have much higher testosterone levels, have a far lower rate of prostate cancer. So more needs to be learned.

Men with advanced prostate cancer are also treated with hormone suppressing drugs – specifically testosterone suppressing drugs called luteinizing hormone-releasing hormone (LHRH) agonists. LHRH agonists are just as effective as surgical removal of the testicles in eliminated the production of testosterone. But who wants to be castrated, either literally or by drugs?

In addition, LHRH agonists present another set of hazards. The major side effect is of course impotence. Then there's the increased risk of bone fractures (researchers found these drugs account for about 3,000 fractures a year) due to the fact that testosterone is necessary for maintaining bone density.(26) Using LHRH agonists may also cause hot flashes (just like a woman, since now the man has no testosterone to counteract the female hormone estrogen – which is naturally present in small amounts in men), loss of mental sharpness and loss of muscle mass and strength. Then there's the fact that LHRH agonist treatment does not cure prostate cancer anyway. The only real "cure" for prostate cancer, according to the traditional medical community, is achieved by surgery or radiation.

If all this tends to frighten you, that's understandable. It's bad enough realizing you're getting old and you can't pull the trigger like you used to, but realizing you may need to wear diapers, be castrated, or even die is enough to make you think outside the box. So here are a number of natural, non-invasive, virtually harmless ways to address prostate problems, including cancer.

11 Ways to Improve Your Prostate and Possibly Avoid Prostate Cancer and/or BPH

The medical community will tell you they don't know what causes prostate cancer. But if we look at the research, we can get a pretty good idea. Dr. Al Sears says,

> If you listen to the AMA, you'd think that every man in every nation on earth gets prostate cancer at one time or another. The truth is shockingly different. Prostate cancer is nearly entirely absent in parts of Asia and some third world countries. But if that Chinese man moves to America? You guessed it. His risk rapidly catches up to the average American born man. . . Prostate disease, in fact, appears to be largely the result of modern technology – toxins we take into our body from artificial foods, from polluted air and contaminated water.(23)

So the first thing to do is to realize that prostate cancer is not an inevitable part of getting old. There are many things you can do to prevent it and even reverse it:

1. Lose weight. Being overweight or obese is really bad for the prostate gland. It increases the likelihood and severity of BPH and cancer. But going on a low-fat diet is not the answer. One study published in the *Journal of Clinical Oncology* showed that a low fat diet did nothing to stop the onset of prostate cancer.(24)

2. Get enough iodine. Japanese men have much lower rates of prostate cancer than American men, and when they move to the U.S., their rates or getting it go up. Dr. David Brownstein believes this indicates that prostate cancer may develop due to a deficiency of iodine, which is much less likely on the Japanese diet than the American diet. Iodine is discussed in depth in the *Complete Breast Health and Cancer Avoidance Handbook* (which everyone should read) and book *Everlasting Health* (see back cover).

3. Get enough sunshine and vitamin D. A study reported in the *Journal of the National Cancer Institute* showed that men with the highest levels of vitamin D were the 17 percent least likely of getting cancer and 29 percent less likely to die of it. High levels of vitamin D were very protective against digestive system cancers (colon cancer), with 1,500 IU daily associated with a 43 percent reduction in the risk of developing such tumors and a 45 percent lower risk of dying of them.(25) Taking cod liver oil is fine, but getting unfiltered sun on your skin is better. Dr. William G Nelson of Johns Hopkins University says that men and women should get at least 1,000 IU of vitamin D (in the form of D_3) a day.

4. Curb alcohol consumption. Too much alcohol wreaks havoc on your prostate. A little red wine (from organically grown grapes with no sulfites added) is OK and may even be beneficial. But other kinds of alcohol are bad.

5. Exercise regularly. Get on the exercise program discussed in the chapter on heart disease in the book *Everlasting Health*. It's a short duration, high intensity program that has been shown to build muscle and lose weight (if needed) better than any other program there is.

6. Stop taking drugs. That includes prescription and over-the-counter drugs. Of course, discontinue them under a doctor's supervision and improve your diet at the same time. Drugs easily irritate the prostate gland and negatively affect your overall sexuality. Antihistamines and blood pressure medications are particularly injurious. If you recently developed BPH after just starting a drug treatment, chances are the drugs caused it.

7. Stop consuming pasteurized dairy and calcium supplements. Reports at the Annual Meeting of the American Association for Cancer Research showed that men with high consumption of pasteurized dairy products had a 30 percent higher chance of getting prostate cancer. Those who took calcium supplements had about three to four times greater chance.(27) This may be because the form of calcium in pasteurized dairy or supplements may impair

vitamin D metabolism, which is important for proper cell metabolism. Unpasteurized dairy is fine and actually good for the prostate. If you can get raw milk, yogurt or raw cheese please do. They are some of the most health-giving foods on the planet. When they're pasteurized, however, they are very harmful (especially to children – see the book *The Truth About Children's Health* on the inside back cover.

8. Stop consuming sweetened foods and drinks. Sugar accelerates cancer and may even cause it (see last section of this handbook). Eliminate sugar and all artificial sweeteners since they are all cancer-promoting, no matter what the media and manufacturers say.

9. Don't barbecue meat. When meat is charred at high temperatures, a compound called PhIp is formed that has been shown to cause cancer in rats. PhIP can initiate prostate cancer and increase its growth. Heterocyclic amines are also formed when meat is cooked at high temperatures when grilled or barbecued, and these are also potent cancer-causing substances. There's less harm done to the meat if you sear it on the outside and leave the inside lightly cooked or rare – the rarer, the better.

10. Don't smoke. Men who have smoked are about two and a half times more likely to have prostate cancer spread outside the prostate (when they get it) than men who have never smoked. Smoking makes prostate cancer or BPH more severe. The more a man smokes, the more likely the disease will advance. Researchers believe that the carcinogens in cigarette smoke promote prostate cancer.[28]

11. Avoid pesticides and added hormones. Farmers (not organic farmers) have a 14 percent greater chance of developing prostate cancer due to frequent handling of pesticides.[29] Pesticides are deadly (that's why they're used) and tend to accumulate in tissues like the prostate. Avoid them as much as possible. Hormones found in meat, poultry, and dairy (added to increase production) cause the prostate to grow. Dr. Al Sears says that being exposed to hormones (estrogens) ". . .relentlessly signals their prostates to grow. It causes feminization, weakness and fatigue and worsens the loss of virility. . . But now men are living longer yet losing virility young than ever. This combination of trends is creating a whole generation of 'avirile' tired old men. And some of them aren't that old. The fast pace of this trend occurring in younger and younger guys is alarming."[30] How to fight these unnatural chemicals? Dr. Sears recommends eating cruciferous vegetables, which contain a compound that when metabolized by the body, inhibits cancer cells.

More Natural Fixes for the Prostate

Tomatoes are good for the prostate. Men who consume two or more servings of tomato sauce each week were 23 percent less likely to develop prostate cancer.(31) Tomatoes (in any form – cooked, fresh, dried, juiced) contain the antioxidant lycopene, which is believed to be responsible for this effect. Lycopene comes in supplement form, but it's best to get it from food. Other foods high in lycopene include watermelon, apricots, and grapefruit.

Cruciferous vegetables (broccoli, cabbage, cauliflower, kale, mustard greens, radish, bok choy, and Brussels sprouts) are good for the prostate. Men who consumed three or more servings of cruciferous vegetables a week had a 41 percent lower risk of prostate cancer than men who ate less than one serving per week. Cruciferous vegetables are rich in a substance called isothiocyates that detoxifies carcinogens.(32) Interestingly, fruit consumption had no effect on prostate cancer.

Cruciferous vegetables also tend to neutralize the estrogenic effect of chemicals and hormones in our food, which signal the prostate to grow. The breakdown of cruciferous vegetables produces a compound called diindolylmethane (DIM), which when added to prostate cancer cells in lab trials, reduced them by 70 percent.(33)

Eating broccoli and tomatoes together seems to have an even greater effect than consuming them separately. Dr John Erdman at the University of Illinois said, "Separately, these two foods appear to have enormous cancer-fighting potential. Together, they bring out the best in each other and maximize the cancer-fighting effect."(34) As part of Erdman's research, he looked at the effect of lycopene, the compound in tomatoes thought to affect the prostate. He found that lycopene alone had no effect, but tomato powder with its full range of vitamins and nutrients of normal tomatoes, were effective. (A good reason not to take isolated supplements. See more on the problems with vitamins and mineral supplements in the book *Everlasting Health*)

Vegetables from the *Allium* family also help cut prostate cancer risk. These include onions, garlic, scallions, shallots, and leeks. A study in China showed that men who ate these foods daily had a 33 percent less risk of getting prostate cancer. China men have the lowest rate of prostate cancer in the world, and these foods are staples in the Chinese diet.(35) Other benefits of garlic in the chapters on diabetes, heart disease, Alzheimer's disease, and breast cancer in the book *Everlasting Health*.

Food for Thought

Tomatoes, onions, garlic. . . Sounds Italian to me. Learning the health benefits of these foods makes it easier to explain (and excuse) why so many people are seemingly addicted to pizza. Maybe there was something about the pizza that causes the body to crave it: The garlic, the onions. Garlic is high in selenium, and selenium is good for your energy and mood (not to mention it helps prevent cancer). James G. Penland, a USDA psychologist found that men who boosted their intake of dietary selenium felt less anxious and more energetic, confident, and agreeable. Another study showed that increased selenium lifted the mood of both men and women.(36) Maybe Italian men are considered good lovers because all the garlic they eat makes them so agreeable!

But seriously folks, selenium could be important in the development of prostate cancer. Larry C. Clark, Ph.D. of the University of Arizona did extensive research on selenium to see if it affected cancer rates – prostate cancer in particular. He stated that taking a modest dose selenium supplement decreased prostate cancer by 69 percent, colorectal cancer by 64 percent, and lung cancer by 39 percent.(36,37) That's pretty impressive. But while checking this research we found the disturbing news that Dr. Clark died at the tender age of 51 from – you won't want to believe it – prostate cancer. That kind of throws a damper on it, doesn't it?

As part of his research, Dr. Clark had volunteers take selenium in supplement form, so it's reasonable to assume he followed his own advice. There are a couple things we might learn from all this: There's little doubt that selenium is important for health. There's research showing that a deficiency of it may play a role in diabetes, Alzheimer's disease, cancer, thyroid function, heavy metal toxicity, arthritis, asthma, and mood. But, taking a selenium supplement is not a magic bullet that will by itself prevent prostate cancer or anything else. As much as we want one little pill that will make everything all right, life just doesn't work that way. Taking selenium, or anything else in supplement form, is a compromise, and may contribute to biochemical imbalances we can never pinpoint or make allowances for. That's why food is your best supplement. Foods have the minerals and vitamins we need in packages that our body understands and can use. So if you want to increase your selenium intake, which may be wise, get it from food. Foods that are high in selenium include sunflower seeds, nuts (especially Brazil nuts and walnuts), garlic, meat, organ meats, and seafood (especially swordfish, tuna, and oysters). But keep in mind that swordfish and tuna have high mercury content, so eat these only rarely.

Another mineral that reduces the risk of prostate cancer is boron. One study showed that men who consumed the most boron reduced the incidence of prostate cancer by as much as 64 percent. They did this by eating boron rich fruits (plums, red grapes, apples, pears and avocadoes) and nuts.(38)

What's more, another study showed that boron can shrink existing prostate tumors by between 25 percent and 38 percent, and decrease PSA readings by up to 88 percent.(39)

Consuming more omega-3 fatty acids has been shown to help prevent prostate cancer from spreading, and conversely, omega-6 fatty acids (as in vegetable oils) were shown to increase the spread of prostate tumor cells into bone marrow.(40) The omega-3s tend to block the harmful effects of the omega-6s, so it's important that you consume enough of them. Conversely, too much omega-6 fat interferes with the functioning of omega-3s, and can lead to inflammation and heart disease. The best source of omega-3s is krill oil, fish and fish oils, nuts and seeds, and grass fed beef. One note on the beef: If the cattle are raised on grain as is typically done in commercial production, the meat has 20 times greater ratio of omega-6 fat than you need and an overall deficiency of omega-3s. So if you eat commercially raised beef, you need to get your omega-3s from somewhere else, and you need to get even more of them to counteract the omega-6s.

Some vegetarians believe that getting their omega-3s from flax seed oil instead of from animal sources is good enough. However, often times the kind of omega-3 (ALA) predominant in flax seed oil is not adequately converted into the required omega-3 fats DHA and EPA, which provide the anti-cancer benefits. This is especially true in people who have impaired health. In addition, a study published in the *American Journal of Clinical Nutrition* showed that ALA actually stimulates the growth of prostate cancer. So taking flax seed oil is not the best way to get your omega-3s. Researchers also found that EPA and DHA help reduce the risk of prostate cancer specifically.(41) So it's important to consume DHA and EPA directly (fish, krill oil, or fish oil).

Vitamin D is also being proven to be important for prostate health and even the reversal of prostate cancer. It's well established that prostate cancer is more prevalent in men who live in northern climates where there is less exposure to ultraviolet light from the sun (that produces vitamin D in the skin). African-Americans whose skin contains the pigment melanin that filters out significant amounts of the ultraviolet rays are also more prone to prostate cancer.

The lead researcher for a study on vitamin D and prostate cancer at Harvard University School of Public Health said, "Our findings suggest that vitamin D plays an important protective role against prostate cancer, especially aggressive disease. This research underscores the importance of obtaining adequate vitamin D through skin exposure to sunlight or through diet, including food and supplements."(42) Men in this study with the highest levels of vitamin D had significantly lower overall risk (45 percent) of prostate cancer, including aggressive prostate cancer.

Consider that normally, over 85 percent of vitamin D is synthesized in the skin due to exposure to natural light. Specifically, vitamin D is synthesized from 7-dihydrocholesterol in the skin (notice that this is a derivative of cholesterol) under the influence of UVB radiation in sunlight. Sunscreens block UV radiation, so it's best not to use them. Cod liver oil (but not fish oil) has substantial amounts of vitamin D and should be included in the diet unless enough sunlight is being received throughout the year. Please see the section on skin cancer in the book *Everlasting Health* for precautions for taking cod liver oil.

There is some evidence that vitamin E supplements may reduce the risk of prostate cancer.(247) However, one study published in the *Annals of Internal Medicine* reported that "Those who take greater than 400 IU of vitamin E a day are about 10 percent more likely to die than those who do not."(43)

There is no doubt that vitamin E is necessary for health and the health of the prostate. But taking it in supplement form is not the best way to get it. Nutritionist Aajonus Vonderplanitz has this to say about vitamin E:

> The worst-case example of a toxic supplement is vitamin E. Most vitamin E is the byproduct of the film-development and film-process industry. Because the chemical waste (tocopheral) is similar in molecular structure to natural vitamin E (d-alpha tocopheral) it is called vitamin E and sold as a supplement. In reality, those manufacturers make profits instead of paying fortunes to the hazardous disposal of their toxic waste. [Similar to fluoride from aluminum and fertilizer manufacturing being used in water supplies.] In other words, profiteers make money by seducing us into purchasing and ingesting toxic waste. Vice versa, foods rendered into waste products after vitamins and other nutrients are chemically extracted, are then made into foods, such as chips and cereals, or animal fodder. . .Even natural vitamin E has to be either heat-processed or solvent-extracted. Heat-processing destroys vitamin E and solvent-extraction causes destruction and low-grade poisoning.(44)

Foods high in vitamin E are nuts (especially almonds), seeds (especially sunflower seeds), spinach, mustard greens, turnip greens, chard, peppers, and olive oil. Since vitamin E is easily damaged by oxidation, exposure to air (keep the olive oil tightly capped) should be avoided and for the same reason, the nuts should be raw, as roasting or cooking would oxidize (destroy) most of the E. Chickens, turkeys, and cattle that are raised organically have higher amounts of various nutrients, especially trace minerals such as selenium, zinc, boron, etc. Grass fed beef as well as eggs from organic free range hens, have much higher levels of the healthy omega 3 fats. Meats, including grass fed red meats and poultry contain little or no vitamin E.[45]

Consuming enough vitamin E will go a long way towards protecting you from skin cancer since it protects the skin from many of the damaging effects of ultraviolet radiation. In addition, those who consume adequate amounts of vitamin E have up to a 50 percent reduced risk of developing bladder cancer.[251] This is especially important for men, since bladder cancer is the fourth leading cancer killer among men, and kills 12,500 Americans annually.

A vitamin E deficiency often results in digestive system problems where nutrients are poorly absorbed from the digestive tract. This can encourage celiac disease (a digestive disease that damages the small intestine and interferes with absorption of nutrients – aggravated by ingesting products with gluten such as wheat, rye and barley), and diseases of the pancreas, gallbladder, and liver. A vitamin E deficiency can also cause peripheral neuropathy, where there is pain, tingling and loss of sensation in the arms, hands, legs, and feet. (If you feel you must supplement with vitamin E, the best brand is *Unique E.*)

David Brownstein, M.D., believes that sufficient levels of iodine are also critical to prevent prostate cancer. Iodine is disucssed in depth in the section on breast cancer in the book *Everlasting Health.*

The prostate gland normally contains one of the highest concentrations of zinc than any other organ in the body. Zinc is a mineral that's helps regulate cell division, growth, wound healing, and proper functioning of the immune system. It's vitally important for the maintenance of the health of the prostate gland, but its exact function in the prostate is still unclear. Prostates that have cancer also have low levels of zinc, and a zinc deficiency increases a man's risk for cancer.[46] But zinc supplements have been shown to not decrease the incidence of prostate cancer. In fact, a study at the National Cancer Institute found that men who took more than 100 milligrams of zinc a day were twice as likely to develop advanced prostate cancer, especially if they had taken it for 10 years or more, compared with those who took no zinc supplements.[47] However, when zinc is consumed as part of food, it is beneficial to the prostate, and increasing dietary zinc is associated with a decrease in the incidence of prostate cancer.[48]

Those on a vegetarian diet are much more likely to be zinc deficient, since the best sources of zinc are red meat, seafood (especially oysters) and liver. Milk and other dairy products have zinc (remember, only unpasteurized dairy, please), as do brewer's yeast, wheat germ, and especially oysters. For women, zinc is needed for vaginal lubrication, which decreases as they age. So women should increase their zinc intake as they age too. Iron supplements will decrease the absorption of zinc, so no more *Geritol* unless you have had a ferritin test, which proves that you are truly in need of supplementary iron. Check with your doctor.

Low zinc levels in elderly men are also correlated with osteoporosis, which makes them vulnerable to hip and other fractures.[49] So it's no surprise that men with prostate cancer also tend to have significantly lower bone density than men without prostate cancer.[50]

The recommended daily allowance of zinc is 11 mg/day for men and 8 mg/day for women. But if you eat the foods you should, you won't need to worry about getting enough in your diet. Zinc is often found in throat lozenges because it's believed to fight the common cold, but there's no convincing evidence to this effect. So don't take those, because the added zinc might add to prostate problems. On the other hand, a large percentage of people test as being low in zinc, and only the *zinc taste test* or an *intracellular zinc test* are accurate for this nutrient. To take the zinc taste test, there's a solution called *Zinc Tally* you hold in your mouth for a minute. If it doesn't taste metallic after several seconds, you're probably zinc deficient. You can order it online at www.thewayup.com. *Zinc Tally* is also a good liquid zinc supplement.

Since it is well accepted that the government's daily recommendations for nutrients are barely adequate to prevent disease and not in any way sufficient to attain or maintain optimal health, many do indeed need more zinc. So seek out the foods that can supply this nutrient and if you take a supplement, do not take doses as high as 100 mg per day or more unless a health practitioner whom you trust has shown you to be deficient with a valid test.

Another food good for the prostate gland is pumpkin seeds. Not surprisingly, they are high in zinc and omega-3 fatty acids. They were used in the early 1900s to treat enlarged prostate symptoms and other urinary tract complaints. One man reported, "When I was diagnosed with an enlarged prostate, a friend encouraged me to eat pumpkin seeds regularly. Three months later, I no longer wake up in the middle of the night to urinate."[51]

Pumpkin seeds have also been reported to be beneficial for improving sex drive, decreasing inflammation due to arthritis, and may decrease the risk of certain cancers.[52,53,54] The recommended amount of pumpkin seeds is a handful (about an ounce) three or four times a week. You can grind them up and sprinkle them on food, or just snack on them. Organic, raw, and unsalted are best. It's best to store them in a refrigerator in an airtight container.

Food for Thought

Here's a tasty salad that will do wonders for your prostate gland. Vegetable ingredients (should be organically grown): lettuce and greens, celery, tomatoes, broccoli florets and/or cauliflower, and onion.
Dressing: ¼ to ½ cup apple cider vinegar; a couple tablespoons of sparkling mineral water; 1-2 tablespoons raw honey and/or bee pollen; fresh ground pepper; ½ clove garlic; other spices if desired. Put all ingredients into blender and blend. Pour over salad. Pumpkin seeds, sunflower seeds, walnuts, and Brazil nuts can be added to the salad - ground up and sprinkled over it. They should be raw, unsalted, and organic if possible. An hour latter, you could have some raw oysters. They're not only going to help your prostate, but your sex drive too.
You'll notice there is no oil in the above recipe since oil and vinegar simply don't mix well, and oil may coat the vegetables, which may impede digestion. Try it and see if your digestion is better. However, if you want to use oil, it's fine, and should do you no harm. Organic extra-virgin olive oil is best.

Another food that's great for your prostate (and everything else) is bee pollen. It is chock-full of vitamins, minerals (zinc), antioxidants, good fats, enzymes, and bioflavonoids. One study reported that men who took bee pollen for four months had a 78 percent improvement in urinary flow, had decreased residual urine and a reduction of prostate volume.[55] A study in Japan reported an overall success rate of 80 percent for improvements in urinary function.[260] Not just that, but bee pollen improves fertility. It's reported that it helps sperm swim faster and last longer – they're more motile and viable. Bee pollen is detail in the chapter on obesity in *Everlasting Health*.

Better Sex for Men Without Drugs

Why are men getting BPH, prostate cancer, and are having difficulty having sex? Humans aren't the only ones having sexual kind of problems – other species are too. Some male alligators' penises are shrinking, so much so that the gators are sexually incompetent. Male bald eagles have decreased sperm counts, and male fish are showing feminine characteristics.(56) These aberrations are hardly because these animals aren't taking the right drugs. They, like us, are being exposed to agents in our environment that are causing them.

A recent USGS (U.S. Geological Survey) study analyzing water samples found ". . . Traces of at least 11 compounds linked to birth control and hormone supplements." These compounds are almost identical to estrogen, and when they get into the male body, emasculating and other things – such as smaller penises, sex reversal in fish, and early puberty in children – occur.

Synthetic estrogens are all over the place. They're not only in many drugs, but in the wastes of drug manufacturing, which end up in drinking water. They're in pesticides, plastics, dental sealants, and some food cans. They're used in cattle and chicken feed because they encourage weight gain, and since the estrogens are very stable compounds, they get passed on to us who eat the hormone laden meat.(57)

If they cause animals to gain weight, what do you think they do to humans who consume them? You guessed it. . .they cause you to pack on the pounds. These compounds are so resistant to environmental break-down, they can survive for decades without losing their biological effect. They're also fat soluble (termed *lipophilic* from *lipo* – fat and *philic* – loving), so they accumulate in fat cells and are very difficult to excrete from the body. They tend to cause an extra layer of fat under your skin, which makes you appear "doughy," and even can cause a gradual enlargement of the pectoral muscles until they resemble a woman's breast. (Smaller penises and bigger breasts do not make the man!)

It used to take a year to fatten a chicken enough for market. Now, with growth stimulating hormones (mostly estrogen), it takes a mere three months. The FDA says that these hormones are safe, but there's no evidence to back that up and a lot to show that they're not. Some cattle ranchers even implant more hormones into the muscle tissue of the cow to get an added boost of hormones. This can cause the animal to have hormone levels three hundred times higher than even what the FDA approves.

These hormones are not just bad for you, they are disastrous to your sex drive and reproductive capabilities. High estrogens levels in men can cause the prostate gland to swell and cause BPH, muscles to weaken and atrophy, make you moody, and encourage weight gain. High estrogen also changes your ratio of testosterone/estrogen, which is an indication of your "manliness." Blood tests can be used to determine your total estrogens (which should be below 100 pc/dl) and testosterone levels (healthy levels are between 650 to 850 ng/dl). Most men should have a T/E ratio of at least 4 to 1. More "manly" ratios are 8 to 1, and sometimes athletes get it to 10 to 1.

(Please note that many health care professionals are using 24 hour urine tests and saliva tests, which have completely different numbers and ranges.)

The more testosterone you have compared to estrogens, the more "manly" and sexual you'll be. So it's important to keep estrogens out of your body, while boosting things that increase testosterone levels. This is especially important as you age because the body tends to produce less and less testosterone – especially after the age of 40. Remember, cruciferous vegetables are very good at getting estrogens out of the body, so regular consumption of them is a good idea.

Other things you can do to limit estrogen exposure are: drink pure water to avoid pesticides; wash fruits and vegetables; avoid processed meats; have regular bowel movements since the longer you wait, the more estrogens are absorbed; eat hormone-free and free-range meat and poultry; avoid alcohol and drugs, since they impair liver function which is needed to eliminate estrogens; and eat other estrogen inhibiting foods such as onions, green beans, cabbage, berries, citrus, pineapples, grapes, melons, pumpkin seeds, squash, pears, and figs.

Testosterone is not just good for your sex life, it protects you from a number of diseases such as heart disease; stroke; Alzheimer's; osteoporosis; Type II diabetes; depression; fatigue; and obesity (especially around the mid-section). High testosterone levels boost confidence, assertiveness, bravery, and valor. Men with higher levels of testosterone are more likely to be in positions of power and victorious on the playing field. Karlis Ullis, a medical director at UCLA says,

> Testosterone is a near magic substance that makes a man a man. There is no other substance on the planet, natural or man made, that can have such profound affects. It can restore or boost sex drive in men of virtually any age. It can decrease fat tissue and increase muscle tissue. It can sharpen the mind and build confidence. It can increase overall energy levels and boost mental acuity.[58]

Obviously, it's imperative for men to have adequate levels of testosterone – not just for a good sex life, but to make it as a healthy, confident, sharp, and manly man. So how do we get more of it? We have to do the things that allow and encourage the body to make it naturally.

High-fat diets have been cursed by the medical establishment and media for over 30 years. But one study showed that switching from a high to a low fat diet actually lowered testosterone levels in men by 10 percent. That may be good news for the makers of *Viagra*, but not for the regular guy.[59]

Testosterone is a hormone, and hormones are built from cholesterol. Fat and diet in detail in the chapter on heart disease in *Everlasting Health*. Low fat diets typically mean the diet is high in carbohydrates, which causes a spike in insulin production (leading to diabetes and the stimulation of the feminizing effects of estrogen) and body fat production. So the first thing you should do to increase your testosterone level is to get off of a low fat diet. Again, it's best to consume fat that hasn't been cooked or heated. Raw coconut oil, raw eggs, raw butter, raw fish and even raw meat are good. Remember to get organically raised food to keep the xenoestrogens down.

Another thing you can do to increase your testosterone level is to exercise regularly in the correct ways. (See the chapter on cardiovascular diseases in *Everlasting Health*) Proper exercise stimulates testosterone production, which in turn increases your sex drive. It also can stimulate the production of human growth hormone (HGH), which is responsible for rejuvenating and repairing all the tissues in your body. One of the consequences of aging is a steady decline in HGH, which results in wrinkles, energy decline, excess fat gain, and loss of muscle tone. However, if HGH is replenished, strength, sexual capacity, and physical function all improve.[60] It has been shown that heavy, gut wrenching exercise can create a surge of HGH. But you need to be in good physical shape to do that level of exercise, and don't do it without proper medical supervision. One of your goals, however, is to get to the point of being able to do really heavy-duty exercises. Consuming more protein (rather than starches) also increases the levels of HGH – so a proper diet is important too. (Remember, some carbohydrates such as broccoli, asparagus and other vegetables are healthy, but starches, like bread, pasta, rice, sugar, are not.)

A common problem with men these days is what's called erectile dysfunction (ED), which is when a man cannot get an erection, or loses his erection at some time during sex. It affects more than 30 million U.S. men, and is more common in the U.S. than any other country. More than one third of men regardless of age may experience it at some time, and more than half of all men over the age of 50 experience it.[61]

That's depressing news: and depression is actually one factor that may contribute to ED. We'll see later that depression is a result of other problems, most of which are physiological and biochemical, so if a man takes care of himself, it will not only help lift his depression, but will help lift his equipment also.

Not surprisingly, almost all antidepressant drugs can cause ED. Many blood pressure drugs, indigestion drugs, antihistamines, muscle relaxants, and sedatives can contribute to it also. (If a guy needs a good reason to believe all along that drugs are evil, this may finally convince him.) So see if you're taking any of these, and consider getting off of them with your doctor's supervision.

One class of drugs that really wreaks havoc with the male libido is statin drugs. Of course, a TV ad shows the football coach all happy now that he's taking *Zocor*. But you have to wonder if his wife is really happy about it, because as far back as 1996, there have been reports of statins – especially *Zocor* – causing ED. Studies have shown that most men who came off *Zocor* were soon able to have normal erections. If they were put back on it, they again developed ED.(62) Why would this be? It's because statin drugs prevent the body from making cholesterol, which as you now know, is the building block of testosterone. No testosterone – no erection.

Food for Thought

Having ED may be a blessing in disguise, since it is often times an indicator of heart disease. Since erections are a result of blood flowing into the corpus cavernosa of the penis, circulation problems could cause it. In fact, arteriosclerosis is the most common cause of impotence in North America.(63) One study found that 64 percent of men who had a heart attack had ED before the event.(64) If you're having some trouble getting it up, it may be a wake-up call to change your lifestyle. You can use the recommendations in this section as a fairly quick and easy test. Try them for a couple or three months. If you see improvement in the bedroom, which you probably will, you may then feel confident enough to try other recommendations given throughout this handbook (and in the book *Everlasting Health* which covers all aspects of health from infancy to the golden years). You may find, that as un-cool or un-technical as natural solutions are, they can make your life a heck of a lot better – for a lot less money too.

Besides cholesterol, another important building block of sex hormones is protein. A high protein, low starch diet will do great things for your sex drive and performance. Red meat is important since it contains creatine, which gives you strength and energy. It's also high in Coenzyme Q10 (CoQ10), which is essential for heart health.

Wild fish (not farm raised), eggs, dairy, nuts and seeds will all help put the fire back in your love life (remember, all are better raw). Egg yolks have all the required fat soluble vitamins (A, D, E, K), iron, and omega-3 fat. Egg whites have all the water soluble vitamins and have what is considered one of the highest quality proteins on earth.

Food for Thought

If you ever saw the first *Rocky* movie, you may remember a scene where *Rocky* (Sylvester Stallone) is training for his big fight. He wakes up, gets out of bed, cracks about a dozen eggs into a jar and drinks them down in one shot. He didn't poach them, fry them, scramble them, or make an omelet out of them – just chugged 'em down. He knew what he was doing, because eating eggs this way – *Rocky Style* – will give your muscles bulk and definition and improve your strength much better than any kind of cooked egg. Forget all those protein powders that are usually loaded with soy protein (bad, bad, bad) and other marginal ingredients. Eat the real thing to get ripped . . . raw eggs. If you think you can't because they're gross, well, just how tough are you?

Walnuts and almonds are the most nutritious nuts, with omega-3s, vitamin E, potassium and other minerals. Others are brazil nuts, pecans, and macadamias. Eating pumpkin seeds and sunflower seeds not only help your prostate, but your sex drive too.

A food that's often times called an aphrodisiac is oysters. Oysters have a lot of zinc, which helps increase testosterone levels. They also help with a woman's vaginal lubrication. Celery is also sometimes considered an aphrodisiac.

Food for Thought

There's a rumor that in order to perform better, male adult film stars eat a bunch or two of celery before they perform. Not just a couple stalks – the whole bunch. There aren't any scientific studies to validate this, but it stands to reason because celery contains androsterone, a hormone that helps reinforce the libido (it's a weak androgenic steroid hormone). Snacking on raw celery and even indulging in a bunch before sex, may make a bunch of difference in your performance. Juicing celery is good and recommended too, but eating the whole plant is also needed for maximum effectiveness. (Of course, overindulging in anything may not be good, so monitor how you feel.)

Almonds, walnuts, pecans or some other nut, and celery are a great sex-enhancing snack. Ditto for oysters and celery together. You'll find that celery helps with the digestion of these high protein foods because it contains a high amount of chlorine. Chlorine (as chloride in the body), aids in protein digestion by contributing to the synthesis of

---

gastric hydrochloric acid. Chloride is necessary for the manufacture of glandular hormone secretions, and helps prevent the buildup of excessive fat, which explains why celery is often times used as a food to encourage weight loss. Don't think you need to eat regular table salt to get chloride, however. The problems with salt in the chapter on cardiovascular disease in *Everlasting Health*.

It's best to get your sodium already in bioactive form from foods like celery. Celery in more depth in the chapter on cardiovascular disease in *Everlasting Health* . It is truly a wonder and is one of the most important foods you can eat since it improves so many bodily functions.

Back to virility. Olive oil raises the estrogen level in women (reportedly without raising cancer risks), which will increase her sex drive. Garlic improves blood circulation – the Greeks and Egyptians used it to improve sexual performance. Avocados contain vitamin E that boosts fertility in males, improves sex drive, arousal, and orgasms. Some say that eating avocados and oranges together for a couple days really revs up your sex drive. Shrimp contains phenylalanine, an amino acid that increases both desire and alertness. Pecans are rich in arginine, which helps hormone levels and sperm counts and keeps sperm upwardly mobile. Even tomatoes (known as the "apple of love,") are packed with magnesium (and potassium) that is calming and helps with stamina.

Smoking constricts your blood vessels, and there's two decades of evidence indicating that it can cause impotence.[65] Caffeine also constricts blood vessels, so it won't help either. A drink or two may be all right, but anything more, and habitual use of alcohol, is not recommended if you want good sex. Of course, exercise is essential for blood flow and sexual activity. Speaking of smoking, celery is thought to be good for detoxifying many of the pollutants associated with cigarette smoke.

Viagra, Cialas, and other ED drugs work by increasing the concentration of nitric oxide (NO – a neurotransmitter) in the blood, which allows the dilation of blood vessels, especially those associated with erections. These drugs work by inhibiting the enzyme responsible for the natural degradation of NO, allowing NO to stay in the bloodstream longer and thus have a greater effect on the blood vessels. (This is similar to how serotonin reuptake inhibitors in antidepressant drugs work on serotonin to improve mood.)

Sounds good, and these pills do in fact work. But one survey showed that more than half the men taking *Viagra* stopped after 3 years because it stopped working. And, more than 30 percent of men find that they had to increase the dose to twice as much to achieve the same effect as when they first started taking it.(66)

Food for Thought

The incidence of adverse reactions for *Viagra* is reportedly small (less than 5 percent). But some of them can be very serious and even deadly (The package insert below which details all the hazards). Conversely, we've never heard of anyone dying from eating oysters or celery. The only contraindication to *Viagra* is the use of nitrates (sublingual nitroglycerin, long acting nitrates, nitrate pastes). Several patients have fainted while using nitrates and *Viagra* because of a drop in blood pressure.

Adverse Reactions listed on Viagra package insert: Cardiovascular and cerebrovascular: Serious cardiovascular, cerebrovascular, and vascular events, including myocardial infarction, sudden cardiac death, ventricular arrhythmia, cerebrovascular hemorrhage, transient ischemic attack, hypertension, subarachnoid and intracerebral hemorrhages, and pulmonary hemorrhage have been reported post-marketing in temporal association with the use of VIAGRA. Most, but not all, of these patients had preexisting cardiovascular risk factors. Many of these events were reported to occur during or shortly after sexual activity, and a few were reported to occur shortly after the use of VIAGRA without sexual activity. Others were reported to have occurred hours to days after the use of VIAGRA and sexual activity. It is not possible to determine whether these events are related directly to VIAGRA, to sexual activity, to the patient's underlying cardiovascular disease, to a combination of these factors, or to other factors (see **WARNINGS** for further important cardiovascular information). **Other events** Other events reported post-marketing to have been observed in temporal association with VIAGRA and not listed in the pre-marketing adverse reactions section above include: **Nervous:** seizure and anxiety. **Urogenital:** prolonged erection, priapism (see **WARNINGS**) and hematuria. **Special Senses:** diplopia, temporary vision loss/decreased vision, ocular redness or bloodshot appearance, ocular burning, ocular swelling/pressure, increased intraocular pressure, retinal vascular disease or bleeding, vitreous detachment/traction, paramacular edema and epistaxis. Non-arteritic anterior ischemic optic neuropathy (NAION), a cause of decreased vision including permanent loss of vision, has been reported rarely post-marketing in temporal association with the use of phosphodiesterase type 5 (PDE5) inhibitors, including VIAGRA. Most, but not all, of these patients had underlying anatomic or vascular risk factors for developing NAION, including but not necessarily limited to: low cup to disc ratio ("crowded disc"), age over 50, diabetes, hypertension, coronary artery disease, hyperlipidemia and smoking. It is not possible to determine whether these events are related directly to the use of PDE5 inhibitors, to the patient's underlying vascular risk factors or anatomical defects, to a combination of these factors, or to other factors.

Special Section:
The Secret Nutrient That May Turn Men Into Tigers

Arginine is an amino acid that has been linked to the release of HGH, greater muscle mass, rapid healing from injury, reversal of atherosclerosis, proper mental function, and increased sexual potency.(67) It's also necessary for the production of NO. So if you have an arginine deficiency, you get a NO deficiency, and you get no erection. Arginine may be helpful in treating sterility in men since it has been shown to increase sperm count, and has also been noted to increase libido and induce erections.(68,69,70)

Arginine plays a vital role in protein metabolism and energy production since it stimulates the enzyme that starts the urea cycle, which converts toxic ammonia (a waste product of glucose metabolism) to urea which is less toxic and which is then eliminated by the kidneys. Since arginine helps blood vessels relax, it may be helpful in treating cardiovascular conditions such as angina, heart failure, peripheral vascular disease, vascular headaches, and atherosclerosis. So having enough arginine in your system is really important. It may not only turn a man into a "tiger" when it comes to sex drive, but help his heart and blood vessels stay healthy too. As with other nutrients, isolated, man-made, or processed variations are not as effective as when they are derived from food, and can even be harmful. Dietary sources of arginine are meats; dairy products; coconut; raisins; chicken; nuts (walnuts, filberts, pecans, almonds, Brazil nuts); and seeds (sunflower, sesame).

Arginine is made from aspartic acid, so having aspartic acid is necessary too. Dietary sources of aspartic acid are meat, poultry, dairy, and sprouting seeds (like alfalfa sprouts). Symptoms of aspartic acid deficiency are fatigue and depression.

Enhancing your sex life naturally will naturally enhance your whole life, without any nasty side effects.

Special Section:
The Common Food Everyone Eats That Makes Cancer Cells Spread

One of the worst things you can put in your mouth as far as cancer is concerned, is sugar. It's a major food for cancer cells. In fact, cancer cells thrive on it. Is this a new discovery? No. In 1931 Dr. Otto Warburg was awarded the Nobel Prize for discovering that cancer cells thrive on sugar.

This is because cancer cells metabolize through fermentation, and fermentation requires sugar. Fermentation is an anaerobic process (no oxygen involved), unlike normal respiration that requires oxygen. So it's not surprising that cancer cells hate oxygen. In fact, a popular alternative cancer therapy is oxygen therapy where the body is flooded with oxygen. Dr. Warburg found that he could create cancer by lowering the oxygen content in a cell to 35 percent and, he could reverse cancer by increasing the oxygen content. (See the chapter on asthma in *Everlasting Health* for a breathing method that will get more oxygen to your cells – and it's NOT deep breathing!) So healthy cells get their energy from oxygen, cancer cells get theirs from fermentation which requires sugar.(71) Eating sugar just encourages cancer to form, and if you have it already, to flourish.

Sugar causing cancer is not just theory. A study reported in the *Journal of the National Cancer Institute* shows that women who consumed a high glycemic load diet (a diet high in carbohydrates, sucrose, and fructose – i.e. sugars) were nearly three times more likely to develop colon cancer.(72)

In a study of 80,000 men and women between 1997 and 2005, those who drank soft drinks at least twice a day had a 90 percent higher risk of developing pancreatic cancer than those who didn't drink them at all. People who added sugar to food or drinks (like coffee) at least five times a day had a 70 percent higher risk of this cancer.(73) So cut down and eliminate sugar, and you'll greatly cut down on your chances of getting cancer.

Another thing that cancer loves you to do is to eat cooked foods. This is again related to oxygen. Cooking destroys not only a lot of vitamins, but it also destroys enzymes. Enzymes are needed by the body for a multitude of reasons, one of which relates to how red blood cells clump together. If the enzymes aren't there, the blood cells will clump more, and won't be able to fit through tiny microcapillaries. This causes many anaerobic (low or no oxygen) areas in the body, thus encouraging cancer. To avoid or reverse cancer, it's best to stop eating sugar (and all starch based carbohydrates like pasta, breads, etc., since they are essentially made of two sugar molecules bound together), and cooked foods. For more on sugar, check out the book *Everlasting Health.*

References

1. Federal Citizen Information Center, The Prostate, www.pueblo.gsa.gov
2. Douglass WC. "Prostate Problems: Safe, Simple, Effective Relief." Rhino Publishing, S.A., 2003. www.rhinopublish.com
3. Ibid.
4. Ibid.
5. www.proscar.com, www.nlm.nih.gov/medlineplus/print/druginfo/uspdi/202649.
6. Douglass, W.C. Op cit.
7. http://w.anniesremedy.com/herb_detail255.php
8. What is the Prostate Gland, www.pueblo.gsa.gov
9. Douglass, WC. Op cit.
10. "Considering Your Chances of Survival." www.pueblo.gsa.gov.
11. http://articles.mercola.com/sites/articles/archive/2001/11/10/prostate-cancer-part-two.aspx
12. Annual Meeting of the American Society of Clinical Oncology, Orlando, FL, May 20, 2002, mercola.com
13. Douglass, W.C. Op cit.
14. Okihara K et al. "Transrectal Power Doppler Imaging in the Detection of Prostate Cancer." *British Journal of Urology.* June 2000
15. ACRIN 2008 Multicenter Trial and personal communication with Robert L. Bard, M.D.
16. National Prostate Cancer Project.
17. Douglass, WC. Op cit.
18. Douglass, WC. Op cit.
18. http://articles.mercola.com/sites/articles/archive/2001/11/10/prostate-cancer-part-two.aspx
20. "Testosterone Deprivation Makes Men Forget." *Science Daily,* October 22, 2004
21. Shahinian, VB, et al. "Risk of Fracture after Androgen Deprivation for Prostate Cancer." *New England Journal of Medicine,* Vol. 352:154-164 No. 2. Jan. 13, 2005.
22. Sears, Al, 12 Secrets to Virility, Wellness Research & Consulting, Inc., 2006.
23. Shike, M, et al. "Lack of Effect of a Low-fat, High-fruit, Vegetable, and Fiber Diet on Serum Prostate-specific Antigen of Men without Prostate Cancer: Results fro a Randomized Trial." *Journal of Clinical Oncology* 2002;20:3570-3571, 3592-3598.
24. Giovannucci, E. et al. "Prospective Study of Predictors of Vitamin D Status and Cancer Incidence and Mortality." *Journal of the National Cancer Institute.* April 5, 2006 98: 451-459.
25. Annual Meeting of the American Association for Cancer Research, April 3, 2000, San Francisco, CA.
26. www.cancer.org.
27. Reuter's Health, May 1, 2003.
28. Sears, A. Doctor's House Call Newsletter, November 13, 2006
29. Giovannucci, E et al. "A Prospective Study of Tomato Products, Lycopene, and Prostate Cancer Risk." Journal of the National Cancer Institute, March 6, 2002 94:391-398.
30. Cohen, JH. et al. "Fruit and Vegetable Intakes and Prostate Cancer Risk. *Journal of the National Cancer Institute,* January 5, 2000;92:61-68.
31. Le H., et al. "Plant-derived 3,3 Diindolylmethane is a Strong Androgen Antagonist in Human Prostate Cancer Cells." J. Biol Chem, 2003 Jun 6; 278(23): 21136-21145.
32. *BBC News,* Healthy Combos Ward off Cancer. Friday, 16 July, 2004.
33. Le H., et al. Op cit.
34. USAWeekend.com, Food, EatSmart by Jean Carper, CookSmart by Pam Anderson.
35. Clark L.C. et al. "Decreased Incidence of Prostate Cancer with Selenium Supplementation: Results of a Double-blind Cancer Prevention Trial." *British Journal of Urology* 1998;81:730-734.
36. Clark L. et al. "Effects of Selenium Supplementation for Cancer Prevention in Patients with Carcinoma of the Skin. *Journal of the American Medical Association* 1996;276:1957-1963.
37. Zhang Z-F, Winton MI, Rainey C. "Boron is Associated with Decreased Risk of Human Prostate Cancer." FASEB J, 15:A1089,2001.
38. Gallardo-Williams MT, Maronpot RR, King PE. "Effects of Boron Supplementation on Morphology, PSA Levels, and Proliferate Activity of LNCaP Tumors in Nude Mice." *Proc Amer Assoc Cancer Res* 43:77, 2002.
39. *Kurahashi, N. et al. "Association of Body Mass Index and Height with Risk of Prostate Cancer Among Middle-aged Japanese Men." Br J Cancer. March 7, 2006 94: 740-742.
40. Leitzmann, MF, et al. Dietary Intake of n-3 and n-6 Fatty Acids and the Risk of Prostate Cancer." *American Journal of Clinical Nutrition,* July 2004 80(1);204-216
41. 2005 Multidisciplinary Prostate Cancer Symposium, Orlando, Fl, Feb 17-19, 2005. News Release, Brigham and Women's Hospital and Harvard University School of Public Health.
42. *Annals of Internal Medicine,* October 2004

Prostate Cancer, BPH & Better Sex for Men

43. Heinonen, OP, Albanes, D. "The Effect of Vitamin E and Beta Carotene on the Incidence of Lung Cancer and Other Cancers in Male Smokers." *New England Journal of Medicine*, Vol. 330:1029-35. April 14, 1994, No. 15.

44. Vonderplanitz, Aajonus, The Recipe for Living Without Disease, Carnelian Bay Castle Press, 2002.

45. Lopez-Bote et al. "Effect of Free-range Feeding on Omega-3 Fatty Acids and Alpha-tocopherol Content and Oxidative Stability of Eggs. *Animal Feed Science and Technology*, 1998. 72:33-40

46. Wu X, Radcliffe J. "Papers on Alpha-tocopherol Intake and Bladder Cancer Risk." Presented at the Annual Meeting of the American Association of Cancer Research, Orlando, FL May 23, 2004

47. Ho, E., Yan, M., *Zinc and Prostate Cancer*, Linus Pauling Institute Spring/Summer 2005 Research Report.

48. UC Berkeley. *Wellness Guide to Dietary Supplements*, www.wellnessletter.com

49. Ho, E., op cit

50. Hyun T, Barrett-Connor E, Milne D. "Zinc Intakes and Plasma Concentrations in Men with Osteoporosis: the Rancho Bernardo Study." *Am J Clin Nutr*, Sept. 2004:80(3): 715-721

52. Smith, Matthew R., et al. "Low Bone Mineral Density in Hormone-naive Men with Prostate Carcinoma." *Cancer*, Vol. 91, June 15, 2001, pp. 2238-45

53. prevention.com

53. Jayaprakasam B, Seeram NP, Nair MG. "Anticancer and Anti-inflammatory Activities of Cucurbitacins from Cucurbita Andreana." *Cancer Letters*. 2003 Jan 10; 189(1):11-6 2003

54. Carani C, et al. "Urological and Sexual Evaluation of BPH and Pygeum." *Arch Ital Urol Nefrol Androl*. 1991, 63(3):341-5

55. Schiebel-Schlosser G, et al. "Phytotherapy of BPH with Pumpkin Seeds." *Zeitschrift fur Phytotherapie* (Germany), 1998, 19/2 (71-76)

56. Sears, Al, 12 Secrets to Virility, Wellness Research & Consulting, Inc., 2006

57. Ibid

58. Sears, Op cit.

25964. Hamalainen E, Adlercruetz H, Puska P, Pietinen P. "Diet and Serum Sex Hormones in Healthy Men." *J Steroid Biochem*. 1984;20(1):459-64

60. Sears, Op Cit.

61. Ibid.

62. Boyd IW. "HMG-CoA Reductase Inhibitor-induced Impotence (letter)." *Ann Pharac*. 1996: 30(10): 1,199.

63. Mirkin, G, M.D., "Smoking Causes Impotence," www.drmirkin.com.

64. Feldman HA, Goldstein I, et al. "Impotence and its Medical Correlates: Results of the Massachusetts Male Aging Study." *J Urol*. 1994: 151(1):54-61.

65. Tengs, TO, Osgood, ND, *Preventive Medicine*, 2001 Vol. 32, Iss. 6, pp 447-452.

66. Rosen RC, Fisher W, et al. "The Multinational Men's Attitudes to Life Events and Sexuality (MALES) Study." *Curr Med Res Opin* 2004;20(5):607-617.

67. Cooper M.D. MPH, Kenneth H, *Advanced Nutritional Therapies*, Thomas Nelson, Inc. Publishers, Nashville, 1996, Pp 87-88, 93, 94.

68. Lamm, M.D., Steven and Couzens, Gerald Secor, *Younger at Last: The New World of Vitality Medicine*, Simon & Schuster, 1997, Pp 62-64.

69. Klatz, DO, Ronald , Kahn, C. *Grow Young with HGH*, Harper Collins Publishers, New York, 1997

70. Hendler, M.D., Ph.D., Sheldon Saul, *The Doctor's Vitamin and Mineral Encyclopedia*, Fireside, New York, 1990, Pp 209-215.

71. www.hopeforcancer.com, www.stopcancer.com

72. Higginbotham, S. et al. "Dietary Glycemic Load and Risk of Colorectal Cancer in the Women's Health Study." *Journal of the National Cancer Institute*, February 4, 2004;96(3):229-233.

73. Larsson, SC, Bergkvist, L., Wolk, A. "Consumption of Sugar and Sugar-sweetened Foods and the Risk of Pancreatic Cancer in a Prospective Study." *American Journal of Clinical Nutrition*, November 2006; 84(5): 1171-1176

Other Publications from *PRI Publishing*

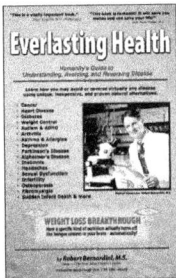

To Order, Call 24 hours:
(419) 869-7901
Fax (419) 869-7935
Email: proreach@aol.com
MasterCard, Visa, Discover Accepted

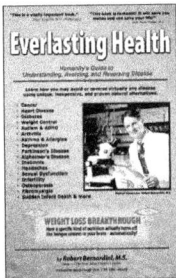

Everlasting Health - Humanity's Guide to Understanding, Avoiding, and Reversing Disease by **Robert Bernardini, M.S.**

The natural health book that dares to break the rules. Over 1,400 references to medical journals, government transcripts, historical citations, and medical text books are used to prove the truth about disease nobody wants you to know. Learn the fundamental flaws in current medical theories, the cover-ups, the lies, and the real reasons people get sick and how to ensure you and your loved ones may avoid and even reverse virtually any disease and stay healthy forever. From infancy to the golden years, this book addresses all ages and aspects of health. Plus how to save money on health care four different ways with complete Resource Guide.
"This book is fantastic! It'll save you money and can save your life!" D. Teplitz, M.A.   *"A vitally important book."* T. Cousins, M.D.
$24.95 + $5.00 S & H   www.avoidingdisease.com
ISBN 978-0-9703269-9-7   6"x9" Quality Paperback, 550

The Truth About Children's Health
by Robert Bernardini, M.S.

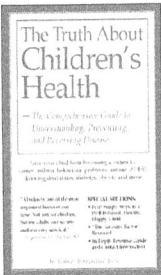

Hailed as "One of the most important books of our time..." by health care professionals, this revolutionary and groundbreaking book will open your eyes to the unseen causes of diseases and how many maladies, even considered irreversible, can be improved and sometimes completely reversed. Heavily researched (over 800 references), it documents how the body and mind of a child or baby differs from an adult's, why this is so important, and the proper steps to take. One doctor wrote, *"This is one of the finest resources on the market. Every parent should have a copy next to his or her bed for quick and easy access. I recommend each and every one of my patients have one and get one for someone they love. This publication is not just informative, but it could save your child's life."* Chadwick Hawk, D.C
$24.95 + $5.00 Shipping & Handling
ISBN No. 0-9703269-6-3
6"x9" Quality Paperback, 398 pages

14 Days to a Safer Child
The COMPLETE Children's Safety Kit

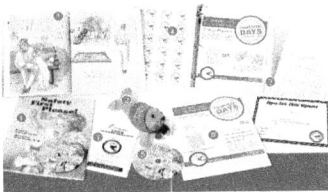

Protect your child to the fullest with the most effective, gentle, fun and doctor approved methods that ensure your child's safety. A 'multi-modal' approach teaches children to recognize dangerous situations and avoid them. For ages 3-12. The kit contains: Full color book, CD with songs and narration, Plush Bean Toy, Parents/Teachers Manual, Daily Lesson Plans, Fingerprint/ID Kit, Fun Stickers. **www.supersafechild.com**
ISBN 0-9703269-2-0
$34.95 + $8.00 S & H